IT'S YOUR HEALTH

SECOND EDITION

LISA DUPREE, MS
MICHELLE LAMPL, MD, PhD
Emory University

Kendall Hunt
publishing company

Cover image and icons throughout text © Shutterstock.com.

Kendall Hunt
publishing company

www.kendallhunt.com
Send all inquiries to:
4050 Westmark Drive
Dubuque, IA 52004-1840

Copyright © 2015, 2016 by Lisa DuPree and Michelle Lampl

ISBN 978-1-5249-0724-2

Kendall Hunt Publishing Company has the exclusive rights to reproduce this work, to prepare derivative works from this work, to publicly distribute this work, to publicly perform this work and to publicly display this work.

All rights reserved. No part of this publication may be reproduced, stored in a retrieval system, or transmitted, in any form or by any means, electronic, mechanical, photocopying, recording, or otherwise, without the prior written permission of the copyright owner.

Printed in the United States of America

Table of Contents

About the Authors . . . . *iv*
Contributing Authors . . . . *v*
Acknowledgments . . . . *vii*
Preface . . . . *ix*
How to Use This Workbook . . . . *xi*
Introduction . . . . *xiii*

Time, Energy & Your Health 1

Vision, Goals & Motivation 7

Stress & Your Health 19

Values, Strengths & Your Health 27

Nutrition & Your Health 35

Positive Mental Health: Flow & Flourishing 47

Sleep & Your Health 53

Physical Activity & Your Health 59

References *71*

About the Authors

Lisa DuPree, MS, ACSM EP-C, CWC, is the Director of the Health 1, 2, 3 program launched by the Center for the Study of Human Health, Emory College of Arts and Sciences. She has been instrumental in the design and execution of this novel academic program. After a decade of experience in corporate wellness working with adult professionals to improve their health, it became clear to her that the time to have set in place healthy habits was decades earlier. Ms. DuPree notes that it has been a special opportunity to engage and empower young adults at a critical time of their life. Establishing a meaningful framework within which undergraduates can set in place healthy lifestyle patterns is a legacy she hopes will continue beyond their years at Emory. Ms. DuPree holds a Bachelor of Science degree in Applied Biology from Georgia Institute of Technology and a Master of Science degree in Exercise Physiology from Georgia State University.

Michelle Lampl, MD, PhD, is the founder and Director of the Emory Center for the Study of Human Health. She and her team are the architects of the innovative, personalized student educational program "It's Your Health." This interdisciplinary evidence-based core course introduces students to the vast topic of health, emphasizing the science of health to enlighten students about their personal lives as well as the broad impacts of health in our world. The core programmatic mission is to inspire a new generation of students to be proactive about their health in informed ways. Dr. Lampl is a physician scientist whose research is focused on human growth and development and includes work establishing the saltatory nature of growth confirming that humans grow intermittently, not continuously. Dr. Lampl is the Samuel Candler Dobbs Professor of Anthropology in Emory College and is co-chair of the University's strategic initiative in Predictive Health. Michelle Lampl received her PhD from the University of Pennsylvania and her MD from the University of Pennsylvania School of Medicine.

Contributing Authors

The Health 1, 2, 3 Faculty team:

Patricia Simonds, MS, RD, Senior Lecturer, Center for the Study of Human Health

Myra Woodworth-Hobbs, PhD, Instructor, Center for the Study of Human Health

Amanda Freeman, PhD, Lecturer and Director of Undergraduate Studies, Center for the Study of Human Health, and Lecturer, Department of Neurology

Acknowledgments

Thank you to the following individuals for their contributions and support without which this workbook could not have been created:

Jill Welkley, PhD, Associate Professor, Emory College of Arts and Sciences for her vision and initial contribution to the Health 100 course.

Shannon Healy and Taylor Werkema for their dedication to the Health 1, 2, 3 program as Peer Health Partners™ and for the instrumental role they played in curriculum enhancement.

Meriah Schoen, BS, Research Assistant, Center for the Study of Human Health, for her time and assistance with proofreading, editing, and design.

Rhea Fogla, current Peer Health Partner™ and Health 1, 2, 3 Program Assistant for contributing her creativity and experience to create the Student Story sections.

Dana Wyner, PhD, Psychologist, Emory Counseling Center, for her inspiration and contribution to the stress and biofeedback content.

Cheryl Wardlaw, PT, MMSc, CFMT, for her expertise and editorial comments on inflammation.

A special thank you to the hundreds of students who have been Peer Health Partners™ over the past four years. Without their energy, commitment and feedback, the Health 100 course wouldn't be possible.

Finally, we thank the team at Kendall Hunt Publishing for making this workbook a reality.

Preface

"It's Your Health" (Health 100) is not your typical health class. This course moves beyond a one-size-fits-all, rule-based traditional health education model. It emphasizes the underlying scientific evidence of what constitutes a healthy lifestyle along with a planned process for developing healthy habits through knowledge application. By exploring the science of health and positive health practices, this course enables students to discover small changes that yield immediate and tangible benefits, at the same time creating a solid foundation for maintaining health and well-being in the post-college years.

The Health 100 course is a part of the Health 1, 2, 3 academic program that integrates evidence-based science education, positive psychology concepts, and health/wellness coaching methodology. The Health 1, 2, 3 program challenges the cultural status quo of health for college students by encouraging them, as individuals, to actively improve their well-being by applying knowledge of physiology and engaging in behaviors that positively influence health.

One of the primary goals of the Health 100 course is to develop a campus community where health is a cultural norm. By prioritizing health, students are inspired to take personal responsibility for optimizing their health and academic achievement.

To accomplish this, the course focuses on strategies that educate and encourage first-year college students to actively engage in achieving their personal health goals. The class stresses the importance of nutrition, physical activity, time/energy management, positive attitudes, stress control, social engagement, and sleep to improve overall health. In addition, the class provides students with methods, including a self-coaching process, to reflect on their health and support developing personal strategies to enhance health and well-being.

The framework of the course combines new knowledge with behavioral change. There are four facets of learning embodied by the curriculum that aspire to:

- educate students in the biological and behavioral elements of health and well-being
- engage students by providing relevant, personalized information on their current health status through self-assessments and other tools
- empower students to identify and make healthy life choices by developing self-management/self-regulation skills
- encourage students to adopt healthy behaviors and habits by aligning current priorities, values, and strengths with health-related goals

Within this framework, students are encouraged to recognize how each content area contributes to physical, mental, emotional, spiritual, and social well-being.

What students have said...

"It was great to be around other students who were struggling to stay healthy in the same way I was and to be able to support each other."

"I always considered health to be something to be concerned about when I grew up, but this class made me realize that I needed to start now and that the benefits will last a lifetime."

How to Use This Workbook

Health 100 is not taught in a traditional lecture format. The way you participate in the course may be very different from other classes you have taken. The course structure is a blend of online and in-class learning and participation. Students are expected to view faculty mini-lectures, access assigned readings or videos, and complete assignments and quizzes online via the class Blackboard site. In class, students are encouraged to participate in discussion and activities that further explore the online content to facilitate learning and application of the material.

This workbook is designed for use in conjunction with the online content in the Health 100 course. The purpose of this workbook is to enhance the content of the course while encouraging critical thinking, discussion, and application in the formal classroom setting. The course Blackboard site and the Health 100 workbook are essential to your success. Each week, you will need to access the course Blackboard site and bring your workbook to class.

In the Introduction Module, you'll get started with determinants of health and the five pillars of health. Each subsequent module addresses one content area and is structured to encompass the 4 E's. Modules may include the following sections:

Education: What's the science?

    🏛 Overview and Learning Objectives

    🔌 Knowledge Nuggets (key pieces of evidence-based information)

Engagement: Why should it matter to me?

    ☑ Pre-Work (things to do before coming to class)

    📖 Student Story

Encouragement: What's working, what's not working, what new strategy, if any, is needed?

    ✏ In-Class Activity

Empowerment: What's your plan? How can it work for you?

☑ Post-Work (things to do after class)

🛠 Additional Tips & Resources

⊙ Study Questions (suggested things to know for quizzes)

Introduction

You are most likely familiar with some of the basic recommended strategies for promoting good health: eating fruits and vegetables every day, exercising to keep your heart healthy and bones strong, managing stress, and getting 8 hours of sleep a night. Often, students who are transitioning to college find it challenging to follow these strategies when they are adapting to increasing responsibilities within a new academic and residential environment. Even with the abundance of health information available on the web, in the media, and in schools, the United States is plagued with an epidemic of preventable lifestyle-related diseases and an overburdened healthcare system. Information alone does not improve people's health and well-being.

Despite the widely publicized risks, over 63% of Americans are considered overweight or obese, and only 10%–20% of Americans engage in enough physical activity to meet current guidelines (BRFSS data, 2011).

Heart disease is the leading cause of death among both men and women in the United States (National vital statistics report—Murphy, 2013). Approximately 7% of Americans are diagnosed with diabetes, a figure that is rising at an alarming rate and is expected to reach one in three by 2050. A 41% increase in the rate of diabetes over the last five years is contributing to a staggering rise in the health costs associated with diabetes. The combined costs of heart disease ($432 billion) and diabetes ($306 billion) account for 55% of all healthcare spending.

Mental health fares no better. Approximately 9% of Americans suffer from depression, with an average age of 32 years at diagnosis. According to the Centers for Disease Control and Prevention, major depression is the leading cause of disability among Americans aged 15–44 years. The World Health Organization identifies depression as the number one cause of illness and disability among adolescents, and considers the rising rates of depression to be a global epidemic.

Many of these disorders share primary risk factors: obesity, sedentary lifestyle, high cholesterol, high blood pressure, dietary factors, and smoking. Fortunately, these risk factors can be modified by behavioral choices. Certain lifestyle elements, such as high stress levels (McEwen, 2008) and inadequate sleep (Colten & Altevogt, 2006), combine with risk factors like poor diet and inactivity to contribute to the negative health statistics. Even though health promotion has successfully raised the awareness about healthy lifestyle choices, we still struggle to integrate these behavioral modifications into our everyday lives. *Knowing is not doing.*

For most people, the deterioration of health is a long-term process. Yet, the emergence of chronic disease and predictors of adult disease are becoming evident at ever-younger ages. Large international studies have revealed that ideal cardiovascular health was rare among children and young adults. The number of ideal cardiovascular health metrics present in childhood was determined to be an independent predictor of adult cardiometabolic outcomes many years later (Laitinen et al., 2012). This information highlights the need for positive health habits and lifestyle choices to be adopted early in life to support health across one's life span.

Many of the lifestyle behavior patterns that lead to disease are cemented in place for young adults as part of a collegial cultural model, including poor eating habits, sleep deprivation, physical inactivity, and ineffective approaches to coping with stress.

Over the years, many students have expressed that college is not compatible with "health," and that's if they think about health at all. The assumptions in place are that to get the most of their college experience, self-care, and health must suffer.

A few of the most prevalent themes include:

- Taking pride in studying hard and partying harder.
- Studying long hours because breaks are not useful and waste valuable time.
- Being too busy studying to eat healthy so eating out of vending machines in the library or late night pizza deliveries become the norm.
- Believing that pulling all-nighters before big exams is necessary and expected.
- Feeling like you're not doing college "right" if you're not stressed out and sleep deprived.

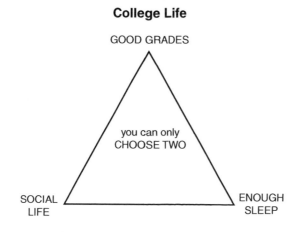

It's not unusual to hear students (and adults) brag about how stressed out they are and how they are too busy to exercise, sleep, eat well, etc. In fact, for many students striving for academic success, self-care seems like a wasteful, even shameful, indulgence. Once established, this mindset and its accompanying behaviors become a standard operating procedure for life's challenges in the workforce.

> **The College Health Conundrum**
>
> How am I supposed to show up to all my classes, study, be social, stay in shape, get 8 hours of sleep, steer clear of unhealthy food and stay sane?
>
> Something's got to go!

Young adults entering college are at a critical transition in life, in which they are developing their own identity and discovering their autonomy. These young adults don't just need to be aware of health basics; they also need motivation, confidence, and support (the *why* and *how* to be healthy). Armed with these tools, individuals have the power to create well-being for themselves and change college health culture, instead of becoming a victim of it.

The greatest opportunity in personal health lies in individual choices and habits. Designing a lifestyle that supports health starts with a foundation of evidence-based knowledge made relevant to the current lived experience followed by application and action. Let's get started by beginning to explore what health is...

What is Health?

Health can be a hard concept to grasp and even harder to define. It is much easier to identify and quantify disease states than health. Health is complex, personal, and multifacetted. It is integrated into life. Health plays a large part in our overall well-being, our happiness, and our success. Health is not one thing. Its complex nature makes it even harder to evaluate where you stand.

The World Health Organization's Constitution defines health as "a state of complete physical, mental, and social well-being and not merely the absence of disease or infirmity."

According to the *Merriam-Webster Dictionary*, health is "the condition of being sound in body, mind, or spirit; especially freedom from physical disease or pain."

The US President's Commission on Health says "Health is not a condition; it is an adjustment. It is not a state but a process. The process adapts the individual not only to our physical but also our social environments."

These definitions have differences, and one would be hard pressed to find someone who completely agrees with just one definition. This leaves us with the question of "what is health?"

Many consider a state of health to be the absence of disease. Upon further reflection, however, many realize that just because someone isn't acutely ill or suffering with a clinical diagnosable disease does not mean they are healthy. Throughout this course, students are encouraged to think of health from several perspectives while exploring what habits are important for creating an optimal state of health.

Pillars of Health

Health is an integration of many different aspects. One useful conceptualization is through five dimensions: social, emotional, spiritual, mental, and physical health. For our purposes, these dimensions are collectively referred to as "the Five Pillars of Health." Each pillar is distinct and encompasses different aspects of the human experience. However, they are interconnected and dependent on one another.

Like the supporting structure of a building, each individual pillar carries part of the overall load. When each pillar is strong and well-maintained, the structure is stable and health thrives. When a pillar is weakened or damaged, the building may still stand, but it is more susceptible to collapse.

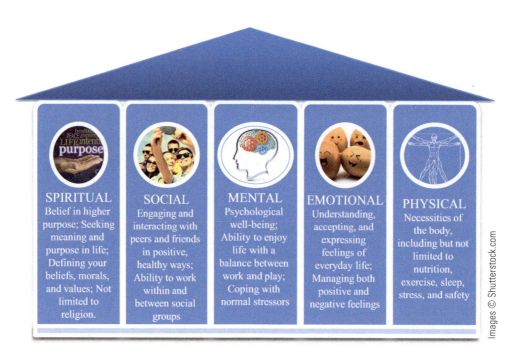

FIVE PILLARS OF HEALTH

Reinforcing one or more pillars or improving the strength and function in a weakened pillar can improve the stability of the entire structure, making it more sound. By improving in one area, an individual is more capable of improving others areas and ultimately able to enhance overall health.

Personal health habits and choices related to time and energy management, sleep, nutrition, physical activity/exercise, and stress influence health in each of the pillars. Levels of fatigue, ability to focus, and how we feel are derived from our subjective experience and often the result of health-related behaviors. In addition, the pillars are not only connected through our subjective experience but also through the physiological responses created in our brain and body. Both subjective and physiological responses can have a positive or negative effect on levels of health in each pillar.

For example, inflammation is a physiological response to something the body recognizes as harmful. The inflammatory process, regulated through the immune system, is the body's first line of defense against an injury or infection. In a positive sense, acute inflammation triggered by the immune system remains in a well-defined area—protecting, defending, and healing your tissues. This type of inflammation occurs immediately after an injury, and is usually short-lived, lasting hours to a few days. Without acute inflammation, dead or damaged tissue would remain, and new healthy tissue would not form.

However, given the wrong information, the inflammatory response becomes a destructive entity, known as an autoimmune reaction. This type of inflammation can become chronic, lasting from months to years. Chronic stress, sleep deprivation, and inadequate nutrition can trigger this type of generalized inflammatory response, which can, if left unchecked, cause tissue breakdown throughout the body. Scientists and doctors now know that chronic inflammation plays a role in many diseases and conditions, including some cancers, rheumatoid arthritis, and heart disease.

Time, Energy & Your Health

"Time is finite and external, energy is expendable and renewable"
—**Loehr & Schwartz,** *The Power of Full Engagement*

🏛 Overview

While people often vocalize their desire to improve their health, many do not follow through. Why is this? A survey of the web reveals that the main reasons people report for not meeting their health goals are "lack of time" or "not enough energy." While life is dynamic and cannot always be planned, time is *not* out of your control. The ways in which we choose to use our time and manage our energy determine our propensity for success. Developing time and energy strategies are essential for ultimately improving lifelong health and well-being.

College is filled with stressors. From midterm exams to career fairs and social events, it often seems never ending and impossible to control. When contemplating going to the gym or cooking a healthy dinner, most of us feel we simply don't have the time. While we may not be aware of it, the perception that time is out of our control can lead to feelings of increased tension in our work environment and an exaggerated workload (Macan et al., 1990). When compounded with other stressors, the inability to find effective coping strategies and regain control also leads to self-defeating feelings and poor academic performance (Papanikolaou et al., 2003). By choosing to avoid the activities that actually restore our energy and positively impact our health, we are ultimately feeding into the stress cycle that seems to be devouring our time.

To effectively structure our time and maintain control, we need to develop a personal repertoire of time management strategies. The primary components of time management include goal setting and establishing priorities. Achieving these goals requires the use of organizational tools and an understanding of whether you feel in control of your time (Macan et al., 1990). Perceived control of time is positively associated with increased job or academic satisfaction, in addition to a higher grade point average (Macan et al., 1990). Lack of time management skills ultimately increases procrastination (Lay & Schouwenburg, 1993) and reduces academic success.

> *"Watching television is the mental and emotional equivalent of eating junk food."*
> —Tony Schwartz

Additionally, research shows that the efficiency with which you structure your time is a large determinant of academic success (Campbell et al., 1992).

Just like health is an interplay of many different components, life is a complex dynamic mix of experiences, people, and time. Life balance is achieved when your time is spent in line with your priorities and what you value most in life. An unbalanced life may be characterized by the "wave of extremes." This wave of extremes often begins with a period of high focus, followed by a swift change to some form of procrastination or distraction. This cycle keeps repeating. Many students find themselves falling into this pattern during the semester. Time and energy management can help students surf the wave of extremes, enhance health, and increase academic success.

Learning Objectives

1. Explore the relationship between time management and academic success.
2. Compare and contrast time and energy management.
3. Integrate activities for time and energy management into the pillars of health.

Knowledge Nuggets

Time management increases perceived control and decreases perceived stress (Macan et al., 1990).

Time management strategies are more effective than leisure activities at buffering academic stress (Misra & McKean, 2000).

Effective energy management can drive engagement and productivity and prevent burnout (Loehr & Schwartz, 2003).

Student Story

Tim arrived on campus as a first-year student, excited to attend the Student Activities Fair, and sign up for different clubs. He wasn't that active in high school, so he really wanted to get involved in college. Tim found many things that interested him and signed up for seven clubs. As the semester progressed, he realized his grades were starting to drop and found himself too tired at the end of the day to socialize with his friends. He started falling short of what was required of him for each club and was constantly stressed with schoolwork.

After some reflection, Tim decided to drop four of the clubs that were the least interesting so he could spend time on the ones that mattered most. He was able to focus on his grades, his friends, and a small set of extracurricular activities by creating a schedule for each week so he made sure to devote time to each. He found this helpful because it allowed him to visualize his week and all the events he had committed to while making sure to allow for some free time.

☑ Prep-Work

- ❏ Watch: Health, Life Balance, Time and energy Management Online Presentation.
- ❏ Read: Chapters 1 and 3 of *The Power of Full Engagement* by Loehr and Schwartz.
- ❏ Assignment: Complete the Weekly Time Schedule, turn in an electronic copy on Blackboard and bring a copy to class.

✎ In-Class Activity: Where Does My Time and Energy Go?

The purpose of this activity is to compare and contrast your schedule to your actual activities, examine the effect of activities on your energy and how your activities fit into the five pillars of health.

1. List as many of the things as you can remember that you did yesterday along with how long the activity lasted.

2. Take out your completed weekly schedule. Compare your list above to your weekly schedule. Consider the following questions:
   - Did you do all the activities you had planned?
   - What's missing?
   - What did you do that you hadn't planned for?

3. Consider the following list. Place a check by leisure activities that you typically engage in. If something isn't on the list, write it in the blank space.

   - ❏ go to gym/exercise
   - ❏ read for pleasure
   - ❏ take a walk/hike
   - ❏ dance
   - ❏ create (draw, arts/crafts)
   - ❏ play video games
   - ❏ hang out with friends
   - ❏ volunteer
   - ❏ going out to eat/snack
   - ❏ watch TV
   - ❏ play sports
   - ❏ play music

4   It's Your Health

- ❏ cook/bake
- ❏ spend time "unplugged"
- ❏ take a nap

- ❏ go on *Facebook, Instagram,* etc.
- ❏ talk with family/friends
- ❏ _____

- ❏ _____
- ❏ _____
- ❏ _____

4. You now have three lists of activities that roughly represent things you should or have to do (weekly schedule, question 2), things you actually do (from question 1), and things you want to do (from question 3).

Consider how you typically feel during these activities and record the activities in the most accurate quadrant on the energy dynamics chart.

Examples of feelings by quadrant:

- Anxious, defensive, or resentful (high negative energy)?
- Burned out, defeated, or exhausted (low negative energy)?
- Invigorated, challenged, or joyful (high positive energy)?
- Relaxed, peaceful, or serene (low positive energy)?

Now, sort your activities into the pillars of health they affect. Note, it is possible for one activity to influence more than one pillar. For example, if you spend a lot of time studying with friends, you may find that while you enjoy their company, you don't get as much done or have as much focus as when studying solo. In this case, the activity would positively impact the social pillar while at the same time negatively impacting the mental pillar.

Physical	Emotional	Mental	Spiritual	Social

5. Looking at the activities by pillar of health, does the activity increase or decrease energy in that area?

Do you have activities in each pillar?

Are you supported in some pillars and lacking support in others?

🛠 Additional Tips and Resources

- There's an app for that!

    One time management app that students have found useful to increase insight into phone usage habits is Checky. Check it out if you frequently find yourself on your phone when you are supposed to be focused on something else.

- Overwhelmed with little things or distracted by time wasters?

    Make a "Not-To-Do List" to help channel your energy into the most important or urgent tasks.

- Not sure how much time to spend studying?

    A good rule of thumb for a weekly study schedule is to spend two hours per credit unit for a lighter class, three hours per credit unit for an average class, and four hours per credit unit for a difficult class.

❓ Study Questions

What is the new paradigm of full engagement in terms of time and energy?

What are the five pillars of health?

Describe the wave of extremes. What does it consist of?

It's Your Health

What is the relationship between time management and academic success?

How are time management strategies related to perceived control?

How are time management and energy management similar?

How are time management and energy management different?

By incorporating time management with the pillars of health, what does energy management work to increase?

Vision, Goals & Motivation

> *"Would you tell me, please, which way I ought*
> *to go from here?" asked Alice.*
> *"That depends a good deal on where you want to get to." said the Cat.*
> *"I don't much care where –" said Alice.*
> *"Then it doesn't matter which way you go." replied the Cat.*
>
> —Lewis Carroll, *Alice in Wonderland*

Overview

You don't necessarily need more discipline to stay healthy or more willpower to change a behavior to become healthier. Having a clear understanding of what you want and need to accomplish, constructing a framework of personalized strategies, and taking meaningful action toward that outcome are important aspects of optimizing health. This module introduces the tools to create a Health Vision, set a SMART Goal, and clarify your Motivation.

Personal Health Vision

Before setting a goal, it is helpful to explore what is most important to you when it comes to being healthy. Creating a personal health vision statement is one way to target what you really want to accomplish. This is similar in nature to a mission statement for a large organization or business. For example, Emory University's mission is to create, preserve, teach, and apply knowledge in the service of humanity.

For an individual, a health vision statement reflects the best case scenario for your health and well-being. It is a bold, desired description of an outcome that inspires and energizes. A well-crafted vision statement helps to focus and guide your effort by creating a mental picture of the target or outcome.

To create your personal health vision, begin by imagining what you and your life would look like when you are at your best—happy, healthy, and successful. Go big and imagine boldly! Your health vision statement will not be the measuring stick for success; that is the job of your goals and action steps.

Examples of Personal Health Vision Statements:

- My health vision is to reduce my chronically high stress level, so that I cope better in my new environment and not damage my health later in life.

- My health vision is to improve my strength and stamina, so that I can continue playing intramural soccer while staying on top of my class load.

- My health vision is to improve my social and emotional health, so that I have greater self-esteem and well-being.

Goals

There is an abundance of scientific studies on the topic of goal setting, motivation, and achievement (Locke & Latham, 2002). Much of the research has been conducted in business and industry to predict and influence work-related performance. Research has also been conducted on personalization and goal setting to influence behavior change for lifestyle-related factors (physical activity, weight loss, fruit & vegetable intake, smoking) (Bull et al., 1999; de Vries et al., 2008; Pearson, 2012).

Research on personal goals and academic achievement highlights a goal setting exercise where the findings suggest that students had a better chance of keeping up with their full course load and improving their Grade Point Average (GPA) with less self-reported depression, anxiety, and negative mood. This study also highlighted that personal goal setting gives more feelings of control, especially in times of transition (Morisano et al, 2010).

Edwin Locke's *Motivation through Conscious Goal Setting* highlights several findings of interest and relevance to health and achievement. One of the interesting findings was the relationship between goal difficulty and achievement. Setting specific, difficult, or "stretch" goals may result in more achievement compared to vague and easily achievable goals. However, certain conditions need to be present—individual ability, knowledge, and commitment to the goal—for greater achievement.

"SMART" goal setting came into use in business in the 1980s where it was used successfully by project managers as a tool for getting results and accomplishing objectives (Doran, 1981). Educators began embracing the strategy shortly thereafter as a tool to help administrators and teachers set their own goals, with the benefits often spilling into their classrooms. Since then, the model has been integrated into numerous health-related behavior change interventions.

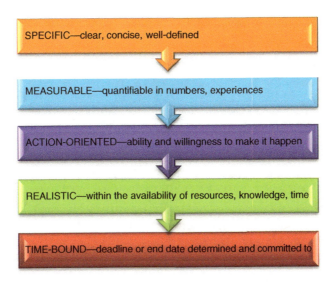

Setting a goal that is meaningful and framed in a positive way along with having the confidence to achieve the goal are also key components to overall success.

Examples of Goal Statements:

Goal: Stop stressing out and being so lazy, so I can get more stuff done (general/vague, negative focus—not very helpful).

Goal: Increase my mental productivity and physical energy, so I can get more stuff done (general/vague, positive focus—better, but still inadequate).

Goal: I will stop using social media on weekdays during the evening between 6 and 10 p.m., so I can get homework done and exercise (SMART, negative focus—more detailed but not as motivating).

Goal: I will exercise with my roommate 3 weekday nights from 6 to 7 p.m. and study in the library from 8 to 10 p.m. on week nights, so that I am able to mentally focus and stay physically active that will help reduce my stress levels (SMART, positive focus—more detailed and motivating).

Once you have created a personal health vision and supporting SMART goal, it is important to identify and understand the motivation behind what you want to accomplish. In his book, *Start with Why*, Simon Sinek suggests that successful achievement of a goal, whether individual or collective, is done by understanding why the goal exists in the first place. This is called The Golden Circle (see graphic on next page).

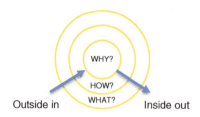

Even though Sinek's concept is focused on business and marketing, its core principle focuses on what motivates us to do what we do. This concept can be applied to many aspect of life, including health and wellness. This circle includes WHY, HOW, and WHAT for doing what we do. According to this concept, most of us start at the outer circle, focusing on WHAT, and then HOW. Sinek explains that individuals often begin goal setting with the WHAT, then the HOW, and finally, the WHY. However, the golden circle reframes the perspective and encourages you to begin with "WHY," which creates an inspired connection to your goal, rather than disengagement. If we can discern and start with the inner most circle, our WHY, we are more likely to end up with greater commitment and better results. Think of the different components this way:

Your WHY is what motivates you, your beliefs and what you value.

Your HOW are actions you take, the process or strategies used to realize your vision and goal.

Your WHAT is your vision and goal, the end result or outcome you desire.

The golden circle is not only a better way to communicate goals and purposes, but it is also biologically sound. The brain's neocortex, which is responsible for logical thinking, attaches itself to facts, or the "what." However, the limbic system of the brain is home to emotions and feelings, and controls "gut" decisions. Decisions that are made because they "feel right," are often those that have a compelling "why" attached to them.

Learning Objectives

1. Explore the relationship between health, motivation, and academic success.
2. Differentiate between a health vision and a health goal.
3. List components of a SMART goal.
4. Create a personal health vision with supporting SMART goal.

Knowledge Nuggets

Personal goal setting may increase feelings of control, especially in times of transition (Morisano et al, 2010).

Research suggests that students who completed a goal setting exercise had a better chance of improving their GPA and reported less depression, anxiety, and negative mood (Morisano et al, 2010).

If you're not clear on your why, it'll take a lot more work to stay motivated. This means you may be more likely to get frustrated, discouraged, and give up.

☑ Pre-Work

- ❏ Watch: Online Presentation—Visions, Goals, and Motivation.
- ❏ Watch: "The Golden Circle" clip from Simon Sinek's TED Talk.
- ❏ Read: Chapters 3 and 4 of *Start with Why* by Simon Sinek, pp. 37–64.

✎ In-Class Activity: Health Self-Perception Assessment and Goal Setting Exercise

The purpose of the Health Self-Perception Assessment is to evaluate your perceptions of health and health-related behaviors in several dimensions, called the Five Pillars of Health. By analyzing your own data, this self-assessment builds health awareness by shedding light on possible gaps to target for improvement while building skills for understanding data collection and interpretation.

How to do the self-assessment:

1. Select your level of agreement for each statement. Circle the number corresponding to your chosen level of agreement.
2. Sum the scores for each statement within the individual pillars.
3. Sum the five pillar totals to get your comprehensive health total.
4. Complete the results section.
5. Use the Individual Pillar rating chart to rate each area's level of health.
6. Use the Comprehensive rating chart to rate your overall level of health.
7. Complete the interpretation and implications section.

Physical	Strongly Agree	Agree	Disagree	Strongly Disagree
I get 7–9 hours of sleep each night.	4	3	(2)	1
I get 30 minutes of moderate physical activity on most days (5) of the week.	4	3	(2)	1
I eat five servings of fruits and vegetables a day.	4	3	(2)	1
I limit my intake of sugar and sweets.	4	(3)	2	1
I pace myself to prevent tiredness/fatigue.	4	3	(2)	1

Total Physical 13 /20

Social	Strongly Agree	Agree	Disagree	Strongly Disagree
I spend time with people that I care about.	4	3	(2)	1
I feel that I belong to a community (social group, club, neighborhood, city, etc.).	4	3	(2)	1
I have someone I can count on to help me out when I need it.	4	(3)	2	1
I have someone who is available to listen when I need to talk.	4	3	(2)	1
I have a network of friends and acquaintances.	4	(3)	2	1

Total Social 14 /20

Emotional	Strongly Agree	Agree	Disagree	Strongly Disagree
I rarely feel stressed out, anxious, or on edge.	4	(3)	2	1
I am not easily annoyed or irritated.	4	(3)	2	1
I am happy and content most of the time.	4	3	(2)	1
I have good self-esteem.	4	3	2	(1)
I find each day interesting and challenging.	4	3	(2)	1

Total Emotional 12 /20

Vision, Goals & Motivation

Mental	Strongly Agree	Agree	Disagree	Strongly Disagree
Even in difficult times, I know that things will be okay.	4	3	2	(1)
I am aware of my strengths and use them to reach my goals.	4	(3)	2	1
I recognize and accept both positives and negatives in life.	(4)	3	2	1
I am good at managing my responsibilities of daily life.	4	(3)	2	1
I am able to balance time between work, play, and relaxation.	4	(3)	2	1

Total Mental 14/20

Spiritual	Strongly Agree	Agree	Disagree	Strongly Disagree
I feel like my life has purpose (sense of direction) and meaning.	4	3	2	(1)
I feel connected to some force greater than myself.	4	(3)	2	1
I find strength and comfort in my faith or beliefs.	4	(3)	2	1
I feel a sense of harmony within myself.	4	(3)	2	1
I use my values to guide my decisions and actions.	4	(3)	2	1

Total Spiritual 13/20

It's Your Health

Results

Enter the calculated totals from above. Add the five total scores to get the Comprehensive score.

Physical score	/20
Social score	/20
Emotional score	/20
Mental score	/20
Spiritual score	/20
Comprehensive score (total of the above five scores)	/100

Pillar	Level of Health
Physical	
Social	
Emotional	
Mental	
Spiritual	
Comprehensive (total of all)	

Individual Pillar Score Interpretation

Level of Health	Range
High	17–20
Good	13–16
Marginal	9–12
Low	5–8

Comprehensive Score Interpretation for Overall Health

Level of Health	Range
High	85–100
Good	65–84
Marginal	45–64
Low	25–44

Interpretation/Implications:

1. Describe your current state of overall health and well-being in three to five sentences.

   ~~Mostly good, a few~~
   On the very high-end of marginal. One point away from 'good'.

2. Do you think that your scores are indicative of your true state of health and well-being?

   No.

3. How do your scores compare with the data presented in class?

   Below average.

4. Do you have room for improvement in any of the pillars? Is there room for improvement with respect to specific behaviors?

   Yes. Get more exercise.

Goal Setting Practice: The WHY and HOW of Goals

Define one goal (using SMART framework) that is realistic and meaningful for you to achieve within a twelve-week timeframe.

My Goal: Do my paper well.

Goal achievement ultimately depends on taking action. But, what decides whether we take action in the first place? This simple exercise will help you quickly discover what is driving you to move forward with taking action toward your goals. The information below will help you feel clear, focused, and more motivated to achieve your goals.

Why do you want this goal? What does it give you?
A good grade.

And why do you want that? What does that give you?
A good GPA.

And why do you want that? What does that give you?
A place in the B. School.

What will this goal help you to do, feel, be or have that you don't have now?
Get a job.

Vision, Goals & Motivation 17

 Obstacles: (What might get in my way?)

I'm lazy.

 Strengths/Resources: (What strengths, skills, and abilities will I draw on?)

I write rather well.

 Support : (What support team and structure will I put in place?)

None, this is a solo mission.

 Assessment: (How will I know if I am on the right track to reach my goal?)

Word count, evidence for ideas.

Taking Action: What is one simple, concrete action that will get me started? Choosing a prompt.

What's the next step? Researching information related to the prompt.

☑ Post-Work

❏ Assignment: Complete Goal Worksheet #1. Submit online in your class Blackboard site.

⚒ Additional Tips and Resources

- Commit your goals to paper.

  Write your goals down and keep them where you (and even better, others) can see them every day. Writing down your goal makes it real. When others know what you are trying to accomplish, it can increase accountability and support for working toward your goals.

- Set performance goals instead of outcome goals.

  A performance goal focuses on achieving something where you have influence over as many variables as possible. This is different from an outcome goal, where success is focused on an end result where you may not have control over all the things required to reach the goal. By focusing on your performance and having control over what it takes to accomplish your goal, your efforts are less likely to be de-railed by things that are beyond your control.

❓ Study Questions

What is the difference between a vision and a goal? How do visions influence goals?

What is the relationship between goal setting and academic success?

Why is a clear vision more effective?

What is the golden circle?

Why does starting with "why" matter for personal goal setting?

What is the difference between positive and negative motivation? Which is more sustainable?

What are the components of academic motivation?

What does SMART stand for?

What is the relationship between motivation and academic success?

What is a gap analysis? What tools were used in class to assist with gap analysis?

Stress & Your Health

"Stress can kill you; it just likes to do it slowly."
—Cheryl Wardlaw, *Taming Stress*

🏛 Overview

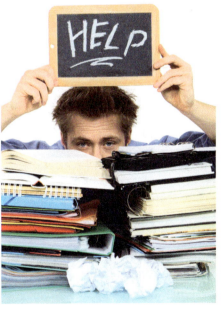

If there is one natural resource, the human race will never run out of, it's stress. You can't see it, and yet, it's everywhere. Stress doesn't have a color, but it makes us feel blue and see red.

Google "stress" and over 500 million results ranging from research papers to personal rants pop up about stress and its effect on us, both good and bad. A certain amount of stress can be motivating, urging us into action, and focusing our efforts. Most of us can think of times when we performed well under pressure, meeting or exceed expectations, and feeling an increased sense of accomplishment and confidence. At the other end of the stress spectrum is when we become overloaded with challenges without sufficient time to relax and recharge, perhaps ending up struggling with fatigue, anxiety, or insomnia.

The 2014 Stress in America™ study found that most people are living with a level of stress higher than what they believe is healthy. It's not just adults in the workforce who are affected, teens in general report school as one of their primary stressors. There is an alarming rise in the number of students reporting feeling depressed or overwhelmed at the beginning of college (ACHA-NCHA National Norms Fall, 2011).

Young adults in college face numerous pressures, and when resources to cope are taxed beyond their limits, the consequences can be destructive. Stress is associated with the production of chemicals that ignite inflammatory processes. Systemic inflammation is harmful because of its effects on cells in all organs of the body. These effects can include altered immune responses, metabolic disturbances, gastrointestinal problems, musculoskeletal pain, and behavioral problems, including disturbances in sleep, digestion, and concentration (Kadison & DiGeronimo, 2004; Lee et al., 2009; Ratanasiripong et al., 2012; Wardlaw, 2012).

> *Stress triggers the release of adrenaline and cortisol. Useful when you need a quick burst of energy, constant low levels of these chemicals can lead to high blood pressure, muscle and nerve inflammation, decreased memory and poor digestion.*
> *Learning to control or lessen your body's response to stress, through meditation, laughter or exercise, has been shown to decrease adrenaline and cortisol levels back to a healthy level.*

Students who learn to control their stress responses within the first year of undergraduate school can fare better academically, personally, emotionally, and socially (Friedlander et al., 2007). In class, you will be experimenting with two strategies for reducing the effects of stress: a biofeedback technique and a meditation activity.

Biofeedback

Biofeedback helps people alter their behaviors with feedback from their physiology. Physiological feedback includes measures of muscle activity, peripheral blood flow, cardiac activity, brain electrical activity, and blood pressure (Schwartz & Andrasik, 2003).

Utilizing biofeedback skills, an individual can influence certain bodily functions that scientists once believed were beyond conscious control. A primary target of biofeedback is the human autonomic nervous system, particularly the sympathetic nervous system ("fight-or-flight" response). The autonomic nervous system received its name because many years ago it was believed that this system operated on "automatic" and was outside of our control.

Through the use of monitoring devices, an individual can become aware of patterns formed by fluctuations in blood pressure, pulse rate, skin temperature, and other indicators of bodily functions. Once aware of these patterns, most people can learn to exert influence over the function being monitored. For example, individuals can develop skills to consciously relax tense muscles or to lower blood pressure.

> *"The time to relax is when you don't have time for it."*
> —Sydney J. Harris, American journalist

Biofeedback techniques have been studied for over fifty years, but the exact process remains to be clarified. What is known is that stressful events can trigger physiological responses such as gastrointestinal problems, high blood pressure, sleep problems, muscle pain, and headaches. Biofeedback, when combined with relaxation techniques, can help treat these stress-induced ailments.

Meditation

Activating the body's natural relaxation response in one way to counter the effects of stress. One relaxation technique that is being investigated more frequently these days by researchers is meditation. There is mounting evidence that seems to indicate that meditation can reduce the risk of depression, increase emotional positivity, and increase resilience to stress.

Meditation is sometimes thought of as nothing more than breathing and relaxing, but the practice of meditation also promotes mindfulness. Increasing mindfulness can improve awareness, helping someone in the throes of a stress response to recognize the physical, mental, and emotional signs of stress. Mindful awareness enhances the ability to recognize and counter unhelpful patterns to enable more positive coping with stressors.

Learning Objectives

1. Explain why stress can be both beneficial and deleterious to your health.
2. Compare the stress response on a psychological and physiological level.
3. Discuss the effects of chronic stress on inflammation.
4. Outline the effects of compassion meditation on stress and inflammation.
5. Differentiate between positive and negative coping mechanisms.
6. Summarize physical, emotional, and cognitive symptoms of stress and methods to buffer them.
7. Define biofeedback.
8. Explore/experience the effect of biofeedback.

Knowledge Nuggets

Stress is a product of a mind and body response (psychological and physiological) that can alter immune response and the secretion of cytokines leading to inflammation.

Stress results in activation of the sympathetic nervous system, causing elevated levels of the stress hormone, cortisol. Intentional activation of the parasympathetic nervous system can help reduce cortisol, helping you feel calmer during the day and sleep better at night.

Research suggests that chronic stress appears to atrophy brain tissue, specifically, the hippocampus, which may affect learning processes and memory (Sapolosky, 1996).

📖 Student Story

McKenzie was a second-year student who was double majoring in Classics and Economics. She had decided to take 20 credits this semester since she did relatively well last year with 15 credits. At first, McKenzie kept up with the workload, and was able to keep on top of the material. As the weeks went by, she started falling behind in her studies. She found herself in cycles of studying hard and pulling all-nighters for a week, followed by doing no work for the next week because she was so burned out. When she was studying for a test in one subject, she would put all her energy and time into it. Consequently, she neglected the work in other subjects, and was left trying to catch up after finishing her test.

The withdrawal date had already passed, and McKenzie felt completely overwhelmed. She noticed she wasn't sleeping well and was having headaches almost daily. She decided to get a planner where she could keep track of all her assignments as well as schedule some much needed time to relax and recharge. After a couple of weeks, McKenzie felt more motivated her to finish her work and continue to take to relax. By organizing her workload, McKenzie was able to stop the cycles of burning herself out. The next semester, she decided to take on a slightly lighter course load, so that she could continue to balance her studies with other activities.

✅ Pre-Work

- ❏ Watch: Online Presentation—Stress.
- ❏ Reading: *Why is Psychological Stress Stressful?* by Robert M. Sapolsky, PhD.
- ❏ Watch: *Stress and Health* by Thaddeus Pace, PhD.

✏️ In-Class Activity & Discussion: Identifying Stressors and Coping Skills

Stress is something that affects us all and can have either positive or negative effects on our health. It is important to recognize what factors cause stress in our lives, identify symptoms, and learn strategies to help us cope when that stress becomes overwhelming. Stress is very much an individual thing: what causes stress in one person may not bother another person at all. Similarly, effective techniques for dealing with stress vary tremendously between individuals.

You will be recording your answers to the following questions in class. There will be a group discussion on stressors, symptoms, and coping skills. You are not required to report your answers if you are uncomfortable sharing this information.

Stress & Your Health

1. What do you find to be stressful? List things that have affected you over the past few weeks. Identify each stressor as chronic or acute.

   Studies take time. Chronic.

   My roommate is very sloppy and his mess creeping closer to me. Chronic.

   Mid-terms. Acute.

2. How do you know when you are stressed? Think about any early warning signs or symptoms that you experience when under stress. Consider physical signs and symptoms (headache, stomach pain), behaviors (snapping at people, snacking, not sleeping, crying easily), quirks (playing with your hair, tapping your pencil, throat clearing), or other "nervous habits."

   When I feel fatigued constantly.

3. How do you de-stress? List your usual coping habits, for example, going for a walk, engaging in a hobby, lifting weights, meditating, hanging out with friends, watching TV, playing video games, social media, shopping, drinking, smoking, etc.

   Play video games. Talk to people

4. How effective are these strategies at reducing or eliminating your feelings of stress?

   Quite.

NOTE: If you have severe or long-lasting symptoms of any kind, see a health care provider. You might have a condition that needs to be treated promptly. For example, if depression or anxiety persists, it's important to seek help from a qualified health care professional. See Resources at the end of this section for more information on services available on campus.

Biofeedback Experiment

Biofeedback is a technique by which an individual can monitor physiological feedback from their body with the ultimate goal of changing it to reduce tension and stress. One of the effects of stress that can be easily measured is skin temperature. When under stress, blood vessels (capillaries) constrict causing a decrease in peripheral skin temperature. When relaxed, blood vessels open allowing blood to flow freely to the periphery, thereby increasing skin temperature. In this experiment, you will be using a small thermometer to measure the temperature of your fingertips. You will measure finger temperature twice, one time sitting normally (pre) and one time after a relaxation exercise (post).

Room Temperature _____

PRE: Hold the bulb of the thermometer between right thumb and index finger.

PRE Temp: _____

Rate how you feel (Please circle)

Relaxed   Tense

0   1   2   3   4   5   6   7   8   9

Describe:

_____
_____
_____
_____
_____
_____
_____
_____

****
Guided Meditation
****

POST Temp: ____96 °F____

Relaxed   Tense

0   1   2   3   ④   5   6   7   8   9

Describe:
___I was very sleepy.___

_____

_____

_____

_____

POST minus PRE = ____96°F____

What did you notice about the guided relaxation exercise?

Did skin temperature change (increased, decreased, or no change)?

What might be possible reasons for this result?

Did your feeling rating change?

What might be possible reasons for this result?

☑ Post-Work: None

🛠 Additional Tips and Resources

- Emory University Student Counseling Center (CAPS) provides free, confidential counseling for students. Website: www.studenthealth.emory.edu/cs/.
- Having a meditation practice can help reduce anxiety and stress as well as improve mindfulness and focus. New to meditation? Try a phone app like *Headspace* to get started.
- Fitting short 5–10 minutes' biofeedback or meditation breaks into your day can help reduce stress, boost energy, and improve mood.

❓ Study Questions

Why is stress beneficial in the short term, but harmful in the long run?

Describe the stress (fight-or-flight) response. What body systems are involved?

What are the immediate effects of stress on the body?

What is the relationship between chronic stress and chronic inflammation?

What are the effects of chronic stress on the body?

What health consequences are associated with chronic stress?

What are some of the physical, emotional, and cognitive symptoms of stress?

What role do psychological factors play in the stress response? (See Dr. Sapolsky's chapter "*Why is Psychological Stress Stressful?*")

List several constructive coping mechanisms. How can using these mechanisms benefit you?

List several destructive coping mechanisms. How can using these mechanisms harm you?

What are some techniques covered in the pre-work materials or in class that help buffer stress?

Explain the relationship between perceived stress and performance (the inverted U curve).

Values, Strengths & Your Health

"When well-being comes from engaging our strengths and virtues, our lives are imbued with authenticity."

—Martin Seligman

Overview

Individuals often struggle with making consistently healthy choices or changing unhealthy behaviors. Often, we strive for unrealistic goals that are out of alignment with who we are and what we really want. This can lead to repeated failed attempts or giving up completely.

Clarifying your core values and character strengths encourages engagement by activating your "internal compass." Setting a goal using the SMART process is a valuable first step for determining which direction to start down the path to successfully accomplishing your goal. Additionally, understanding your "why" through the golden circle allows you to develop an inspired SMART goal that connects with your personal health vision statement. However, knowing the values that are attached to *why* you want to go for that particular goal and *how* to get there are often neglected when mapping out the route to your desired destination. If you clearly understand your values and utilize your character strengths, you are more likely to make sure your actions bring you closer to that destination each and every day.

This week in class, you will identify how to use your values and strengths in everyday life and integrate these foundational elements into your SMART health goal through the creation of supporting action steps.

Values

Identifying and exploring values seeks to delve deeper into the question "Why is this goal important to you?"

A value is something that has intrinsic merit. Values are principles or standards of behavior that you judge to be important or right. Think of values as part of your internal compass. Your values are reflected in your behavior on a day-to-day basis. The values you identify with help guide your decisions, choices, and behaviors.

Interestingly, researchers have begun to look at values not only from a psychological perspective, but a physiological one also. Research on personal values and stress response indicates that affirming values coupled with dispositional strong self-resources (e.g., self-esteem and optimism) had a protective effect against psychological reactions to stressful events. In addition, individuals in a value-affirming group had a buffered neuroendocrine response to stress; specifically, a lower cortisol response (Creswell et al., 2005). This finding implies that there was less activation of the fight-or-flight response to stress. The fight-or-flight response is a natural reaction that is only meant to be triggered occasionally. However, modern living keeps tripping it, sending the response into overdrive. Chronic activation of this chemical cascade is implicated as a factor in stress, anxiety, depression, and other health problems.

Character Strengths

You may be familiar with the old saying "play to your strengths." In recent years, research in the field of positive psychology has been providing the scientific underpinnings for the importance of character strengths and the benefits resulting from strength use.

Research on character strengths, well-being, and quality of life by Linley, Maltby, and Proctor (2011) suggests that strength use is positively correlated with individual sense of self, self-esteem, and self-efficacy as well as well-being and health-related quality of life. Furthermore, some strengths, specifically hope, zest, gratitude, love, and curiosity, are associated with overall life satisfaction (Park, Peterson, & Seligman, 2004).

Character strengths are different from other types of strengths, like talent (the ability to do something well), interests (things we enjoy doing), skills (proficiencies we develop), and resources (external support) (Niemeic, 2014, p. 26). They allow us to display our virtues and human goodness by reflecting our identity and authentic selves.

Signature strengths are those that come forth naturally in many different situations. As they are core to identity, signature character strengths powerfully affect decisions, preferences, and actions.

When we express our signature strengths, we feel alive and energized. We experience pleasure, engagement, and meaning in our lives. Intentionally utilizing them in our close relationships, communities, academics, and health behavior can be deeply satisfying. For these reasons, strengths may help provide a directional compass for determining how to take steps to move further down the path for reaching our goals.

Transition is an excellent time to explore values and strengths. Identifying what is really important and appreciating your innate abilities is a fulfilling way to navigate the path toward your goals during times of change. Aligning health goals and supporting actions with values and strengths have the potential to generate great "aha" moments, empowering you to actively stay healthy.

Learning Objectives

1. Define values and understand how to use them for health improvement.
2. Describe how value affirmation may affect stress and health.
3. Identify the relationship between character strength use and success in various aspects of life.
4. Identify your core values and signature strengths and how you have used them.
5. Create action steps for your health goal that support your top values and utilize your strengths.

Knowledge Nuggets

Research on personal values and stress response indicated that affirming values coupled with strong self-resources had a protective effect against psychological reactions to stressful events. Individuals in the value-affirming group had a buffered neuroendocrine response to a stress event; specifically, a lower cortisol response (Creswell et al., 2005).

People who use their strengths more have higher levels of energy, experience less stress, are more likely to achieve their goals and perform better at work (Corporate Leadership Council Performance Management Survey, 2002; Govindji & Lindley, 2007; Linley et al., 2010; Wood et al., 2011).

Interventions that improve psychological well-being and self-control could promote healthy weight loss by focusing on higher values rather than immediate impulses and stressors (Logel & Cohen, 2012)

Pre-Work

- ❏ Watch: Online Presentation—Values and Strengths.
- ❏ Reading: *Mind the Gap: Cultivating Change and Closing the Disengagement Divide* by Brené Brown.
- ❏ Assignment: VIA Character Strengths Survey—complete before class, record your top five strengths. You will be using these to complete the homework for this week.

Top five character strengths

1.
2.
3.
4.
5.

✏️ In-Class Activity: Values Discussion and Strengths Integration

Discussion questions:

1. In the reading for this week, Dr. Brown describes a disengagement divide as a gap between practiced and aspirational values. Do you think Emory has a culture of "never enough" or "success at any cost"?
2. How might a culture of "success at any cost" affect health?
3. Think about a recent personal example in which you demonstrated the disengagement divide. Why was it difficult to achieve your aspirational value?
4. How could "minding the gap" lead us toward a culture shift? What can we do individually to practice "minding the gap"?

Character Strengths Goal Integration Exercise

Purpose: To explore ways to use character strengths by creating actions steps for a health-related goal based on a sample student scenario and their signature character strengths.

Instructions: Working in small groups, brainstorm multiple answers to the following questions for each of the identified character strengths given a specific scenario.

Each group will have a chance to "be the voice" for the student in the scenario and share how they would answer the questions.

For your scenario, answer the following questions for the character strengths listed.

1. What might be a goal or priority of someone in this situation?
2. Consider how a person in this situation might use each of their strengths. What is a specific strength-based action that this person could take that supports their goal or priority (from question 1)?

Scenario 1: You are a new student on campus who doesn't know anyone. The transition into a new environment has been stressful and you want to develop a support network.

Your top three character strengths are:

1. Love of learning
2. Leadership
3. Self-regulation

Goal or priority: _____

Strengths based Actions Steps:

1. _____
2. _____
3. _____

Scenario 2: You are enrolled in a class where a significant part of your grade is determined by a group project. You are assigned to a group with four other peers. Two of your group members are not contributing their best effort to the project.

Your top three character strengths are:

1. Zest
2. Judgment and open-mindedness
3. Creativity

Goal or priority: _Getting everybody to contribute equally._

Strengths based Actions Steps:

1. _Using (1) to motivate and energize._
2. _Using (2) to see if there is a good reason._
3. _Using (3) to find a way to apply their strengths._

Scenario 3: You are living in a dorm and have a roommate for the first time in your life. You and your roommate get along pretty well but lately your roommate has started coming in late at night and waking you up. This is causing a conflict between the two of you.

Your top three character strengths are:

1. Humor
2. Prudence and discretion
3. Curiosity

Goal or priority: _____

Strengths based Actions Steps:

1. _____
2. _____
3. _____

Scenario 4: You are excited about all the different opportunities available on campus and want to make the most of your time in college. You are interested in joining an organization or club on campus, but tend to shy away from unfamiliar situations where you don't know anyone.

Your top three character strengths are:

1. Appreciation of beauty and excellence
2. Perspective
3. Kindness

Goal or priority: _____

Strengths based Actions Steps:

1. _____
2. _____
3. _____

Scenario 5: You have been offered a position as a team leader for a group on campus. This is a new experience for you, but you are ready to take on the challenge.

Your top three character strengths are:

1. Modesty and humility
2. Gratitude
3. Social intelligence

Goal or priority: _____

Strengths based Actions Steps:

1. _____
2. _____
3. _____

Adapted from Froh, J. J., & Parks, A. *Activities for Teaching Positive Psychology: A Guide for Instructors*, Ch. 3, pp. 23–28. Washington, DC: American Psychological Association, 2013.

Personal Application Practice: Consider something you want to improve or a specific difficulty that you've experienced during the transition into your first semester in college.

Goal or priority: _____

Your top three character strengths are:

1. _____
2. _____
3. _____

Strengths based Actions Steps:

1. _____
2. _____
3. _____

☑ Post-Work

❏ Assignment: Complete Goal Worksheet #2 and submit online.

✹ Additional Tips and Resources

- Strength Spotting—Become more aware of how and when you use your strengths. Pick an ordinary day and set your phone or alarm to signal you each hour. When you hear the alarm, stop and notice what you are doing and which strength you are using. Keep a log for the day. At the end of the day, look back to see your strengths use and if there are any patterns.

- Learn more about Character Strengths:

  Character Strengths YouTube channel: www.youtube.com/VIAstrengths.

- "Affirmation of Personal Values Buffers Neuroendocrine and Psychological Response to Stress." *Psychological Science* 16.11 (2005): 846–851.

It's Your Health

❓ Study Questions

What are values? How do they influence health?

What is the relationship between value affirmation, stress, and health goals?

What are strengths? How do they influence health? Why might it be beneficial to focus on your strengths rather than your flaws?

What is the relationship between strengths use, grade point average, life satisfaction, and college satisfaction?

What benefits might you see from incorporating your values and strengths into your action steps? How might this influence your goal success?

What are practiced values?

What are aspirational values?

What is the disengagement divide?

Honesty
Judgment
Bravery
Spirituality
Curiosity

Nutrition & Your Health

"Let food be thy medicine, and medicine be thy food"
—Hippocrates

Overview

Foods play an important role in our health, for both good and bad. The health benefits of food can be extraordinary, and offer a simple way for each of us to take care of ourselves and improve our health. Few people, however, contemplate their health each time they sit down for a meal. We eat based on "what we feel like" at the time. Sometimes we choose whatever is fast. Other times, we eat based on calories, price, desire to feel full, or simply the way our families ate. A fundamental challenge is that while we eat many items, not everything we consume is able to meet the body's nutritional needs. We eat for many reasons beyond nourishment—for pleasure, out of boredom (for "something to do"), to self-sooth in times of stress, and as an opportunity for social interaction. Becoming aware of our eating habits and learning to think about our food choices as health opportunities are important steps toward improving our health and well-being.

Each time we pick up a fork or munch on a snack, we have an opportunity to both fuel our bodies and enhance our health. From an early age, we are taught about the importance of eating three primary macronutrients: protein, fat, and carbohydrates. When consumed in a balanced manner, these nutrients maintain the health and functionality of our bodies. In contrast to the way diets are conveyed on the Internet, in magazines, and other popular media, there is not merely one "correct" eating pattern through which we can attain the proper balance of these macronutrients. Instead, there are numerous foods that provide protein, carbohydrates, and fat, and it is our unique taste preferences that determine how we navigate these options.

With so much conflicting nutrition information, it can be difficult to decide which food options promote health. Often misinformation is advertised by companies with a vested interest in convincing us to purchase their food, products, or dietary supplements. "Low-fat! No sugar added! High fiber! No trans fats!"... these types of labels lead us to believe that these products are a good way to gain important nutrients, and avoid things that are bad for us. The concepts of "good" and "bad" foods are both fluid and unique for everyone. The best way to ensure that we are nourishing our bodies is to eat whole foods, which provide a rich mix of macro- and micronutrients. Nutritional supplements, while often seen as an easier solution, generally do not provide the natural forms of vitamins and minerals. And, the nutrients are absorbed less effectively than those found in whole foods.

Beyond eating whole foods, it is essential that our diet contains a wide variety of fruits and vegetables. In addition to being nutrient-dense, many fruits and vegetables also contain phytonutrients. These are chemicals that provide color, odor, and flavor to plants, and often contain potent anti-inflammatory effects. As inflammation is a common link between diabetes, cardiovascular disease, and cancer (which account for almost 70% of all deaths in the United States [Kiecolt-Glaser, 2010]), what and how we are currently eating is killing us. By choosing brightly colored fruits and vegetables, we are ingesting chemicals that can directly decrease inflammation and increase our resistance to stress in our cells (Howitz & Sinclair, 2008). In this way, nutrition can be our first line of defense against the negative physical effects of chronic stress and inflammation.

This is in contrast to a diet rich in added sugars, red meat, trans fats, fried foods, and refined grains, which is a hallmark of the standard American or "Western" diet. The consumption of these foods actually promotes a constant pro-inflammatory state in our bodies, increasing our risks of both physical diseases and depression (Manosso, Moretti, Rodrigues, 2013; Kiecolt-Glaser, 2010). It would be difficult to completely remove these food items from our diet, however, we can enhance our intake of fruits and vegetables while still enjoying unhealthier foods in moderation. Like many other things in life, a healthy diet is not an all or nothing proposition. Adopting a flexitarian approach can help us make positive changes while maintaining the flexibility in food choices that we desire. With a focus on increasing plant-based foods and reducing highly processed foods (Raphaely et al., 2013), this eating style enhances healthy habits known to decrease inflammation and lower the risk for diabetes and heart disease (Brunner et al., 2008). While a flexitarian diet does not represent a single dietary pattern or experience, it suggests that even small changes in diet can have long-term beneficial health effects.

Making the transition to eating at college can be challenging. Unfamiliar foods, prepared in different ways, located in unusual facilities, amid strangers, and available 24/7 can lead to some unhealthy choices. In this module, we will introduce the importance of food for nutrition and health, with an emphasis on its relationship to inflammation, and offer some guidance on how to find and make healthy choices here on Emory's campus.

Inflammation is kept local and appropriate by taking in key nutrients, such as Omega 3, and anti-oxidants. Foods rich in Omega 3 include grass-fed beef, cold-water wild-caught fish, ground flax seeds, and walnuts. Colorful fruits and vegetables are excellent sources of anti-oxidants.

Nutrition & Your Health

Learning Objectives

1. Identify your personal eating behaviors.
2. Explain the relationship between eating behaviors, stress and inflammation.
3. Discuss how specific phytonutrients benefit your health.
4. Design healthy meals and snacks based on anti-inflammatory foods that you can consume on a daily basis.

Knowledge Nuggets

Stress can influence our eating behaviors.

Choosing anti-inflammatory foods is a powerful tool in protecting your body against the effects of chronic stress-induced inflammation. These effects include not only increased risk of chronic physical diseases but susceptibility to depression (Manosso et al., 2003; Kiecolt-Glaser, 2010)

Brightly colored fruits and vegetables contain powerful chemical compounds called phytonutrients that can decrease inflammation and increase resistance to stress in your cells (Howitz & Sinclair, 2008).

Student Story

After coming to college, Matt's eating habits changed a lot compared to how he ate at home. He had the unlimited swipes meal plan and ate exclusively burgers, fries, and pizza at the Dobbs University Center (DUC). He didn't like salad so he avoided the salad bar, and whenever he goes to the DUC at lunchtime, the sandwich line was too long for him to wait in. Every time he headed out of the DUC, he grabbed some ice cream to go. After a few weeks, Matt was feeling sluggish throughout the entire day and had no energy to do work.

He decided to try a new strategy with eating. He started to try the Vegan, Comfort, and Global sections more often and would occasionally have a burger and fries. If he were still feeling hungry after eating, he would grab an apple or banana on the way out rather than getting ice cream. Matt realized that a gradual shift to a variety of more nutritious foods was a good approach for him because he noticed he began to have more energy and focus throughout the day.

Pre-Work (checklist)

- ❏ Watch: Online Presentation.
- ❏ Read: Chapter 3 of *In Defense of Foods* by Michael Pollan.
- ❏ Watch video: "Appropriating Plant Defenses" by Michael Greger M.D.
- ❏ Assignment: Photo Plate: take a photo of one meal you consume this week. Submit the photo in the class Blackboard site and bring a copy to class to use for the in-class activity.

It's Your Health

✏️ In-Class Activity

This week in class, you will complete your photo plate evaluation using the "meal photo plate" that you brought to class. You will also complete a 24-hour food recall to evaluate fruit and vegetable intake.

1. Review and compare the "meal photo plate" with the reference plates provided in class. What do you notice about the comparison? Are there any sections of the plate missing?

    Missing vegetables.

2. List the food items on the plate in your photo and which macronutrients they each provide (carbohydrates, protein, and fat).

    Carbs, proteins, fats, vitamins

3. Review the plate for color. What colors did you consume? Did anyone color dominate the plate?

    All but green. Red.

4. What about your plate do you consider to be a healthy?

    Fruit.

5. What can you easily add/remove to increase the potential health benefits of this plate?

    Add vegetables.

6. In the space provided below record a 24-hour recall of all the food that you consumed yesterday.

    Pizza. Chicken. Fruit. Pasta. Rice. Beef. Water, Tea. Tofu.

    AI   AI   AI

7. Using the fruit and vegetable tracking sheet (Figure 1), record your intake of fruits and vegetables for the day. Answer the question for each color category.

Nutrition & Your Health

8. Examine the charts of phytonutrients (Figure 2a and 2b) and identify which phytonutrients you have consumed and how these promote specific health effects.

9. Examine the chart of Anti-Inflammatory Fats & Proteins (Figure 3), Anti-Inflammatory Drinks (Figure 4), and Anti-Inflammatory Spices & Herbs (Figure 5). Identify any that you have consumed.

☑ Post-Work: None

✗ Additional Tips & Resources

- Incorporate plants with each meal throughout the day.

  Try adding spinach in with your eggs or into a smoothie for an easy vegetable addition to breakfast. Choosing to start the day with a vegetable or fruit helps to increase overall consumption of phytonutrients.

- Eat real food.

  Refined or processed foods tend to be bland in colors unless artificially colored. Reading food labels helps to increase awareness of artificial colors and dyes that might be used in a product along with preservatives or other unnecessary ingredients.

- Combine macronutrients protein, carbohydrates, and fats within each meal to promote balance. This will help maintain blood sugar levels and satiety while promoting more variety of nutrients consumed. An example of this would be to have a slice of whole grain bread with banana and peanut butter.

❓ Study Questions

What are the health risks of the standard "American" diet?

Describe the relationship between stress and eating.

List ways in which diet can be both a positive and negative influence.

Evaluate what makes foods unhealthy.

Why do you need to eat phytonutrients?

Why do nutrients in pill form not replace food?

How many fruits & vegetables did you consume yesterday?

Place a check in the box next to each color you consumed and total them up at the bottom. Examples of colors are provided. *Note, not all fruits and vegetables are listed here.

Color						What can you add to your consumption?
RED Strawberries Pomegranates Tomato Apples Kidney beans Beans Red bell pepper Watermelon	✓					What can you add to your consumption in the red category?
ORANGE Butternut squash Orange Sweet potato Orange bell pepper Apricot Carrots	✓					What can you add to your consumption in the orange category?
YELLOW Corn Popcorn Lemon Spaghetti squash Yellow squash Yellow bell pepper Banana						What can you add to your consumption in the yellow category?
GREEN Broccoli Bell peppers Avocado Brussel sprouts Greens Kale Cabbage Apples Grapes Celery Cucumber Lettuce	✓	✓				What can you add to your consumption in the green category?
BLUE/PURPLE Blueberries Grapes Eggplant Dates Raisins Varieties of "purple": Potatoes, Carrots, Cabbage, Kale						What can you add to your consumption in the blue/purple category?
TAN/WHITE Onions Hummus Nuts Seeds Tahini Garlic	✓					What can you add to your consumption in the tan category?
Total Fruit & Vegetable Consumption						

Figure 1

Green

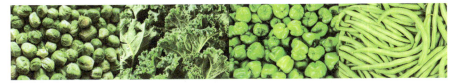

Supports eye, lung, and cell health; Enhances arterial function; Aids with wound healing

Red

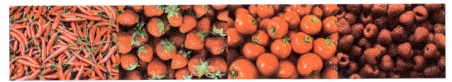

Supports Prostate and Urinary Tract Health; Protects against cancer and heart disease

Purple/Blue

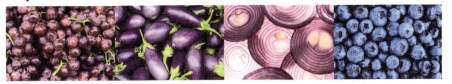

Supports brain, bone, heart, arterial, and cognitive health; Protects against cancer and aging

Orange/Yellow

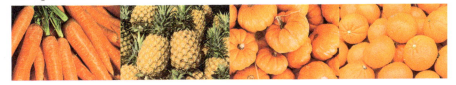

Supports eye and immune health; Aids in healthy growth and development

White

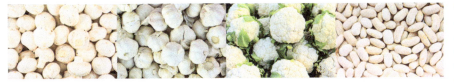

Supports bone, arterial, and circulatory system health; Protects against heart disease and cancer

Figure 2a
All images © Shutterstock, Inc.

Phytochemical	Food Source	Health Benefit
Allicin	Garlic, onion, leeks, chives	Act as an antioxidant and antimicrobial; lower blood pressure and cholesterol
Anthocyanins	Blueberries, blackberries, red apples, red potatoes, black raspberries, black currants, gooseberries	Act as antioxidants; lower blood pressure, improve vision, protect against cancer and heart disease, reduce inflammation
Capsaicin	Chili peppers	Lower blood pressure, lower cholesterol, reduce inflammation, prevent blood clots
Carotenoids	Carrots, sweet potatoes, pumpkins, apricots, peaches, tomatoes, brightly colored peppers, dark leafy green vegetables	Act as antioxidants; reduce risk of cancer and heart disease, enhance immune response
Flavonoids	Onions, curly kale, broccoli, apples, blueberries, purple grapes, whole wheat, red wine, dark chocolate, tea	Act as antioxidants; Reduce risk of heart disease, protect against peptic ulcers, anti-cancer, reduce inflammation
Isoflavones	Soy products and legumes	Reduce risk of breast, colon, prostate, and ovarian cancer; reduce risk of osteoporosis
Indoles	Cruciferous vegetables: Brussels sprouts, broccoli, cabbage, cauliflower, horseradish, mustard greens, kale, turnip greens	May inhibit action of estrogen and reduce risk of cancer
Lignans	Flaxseed, sesame seed, whole grains (rye, wheat, oat, barley), soy beans, cruciferous vegetables, apricots, strawberries, nuts, seeds	Reduce risk of breast, ovarian, prostate, and colon cancer; reduce risk of heart disease
Phenolic Acids	Tea, coffee, berries, oranges, pears, prunes, soybeans, oats, potatoes	Protect against oxidative damage, heart disease, stroke, cancer
Resveratrol	Grapes, wine, grape juice, peanuts, blueberries, cranberries	Prevents damage to blood vessels and blood clots, reduce LDL cholesterol
Tannins	Grapes, persimmons, lentils, blueberries, tea, chocolate, wine	Act as antioxidants, reduce risk of cancer

Figure 2b

Anti-inflammatory Fats & Proteins

High Quality Natural Cheese

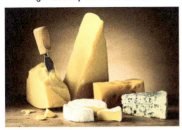

High Quality Yogurt

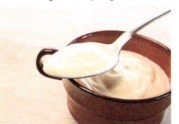

Omega-3 Enriched Eggs

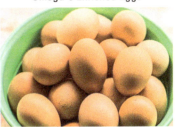

Skinless Chicken Breast

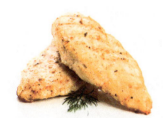

Lean Grass-Fed Meats

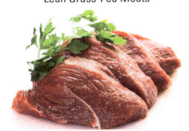

Fish/Seafood Rich in Omega-3: Salmon, herring, sardines, black cod

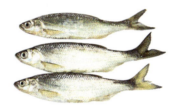

Quinoa

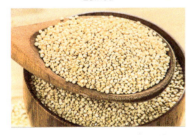

Low Fat or Fat Free Cottage Cheese

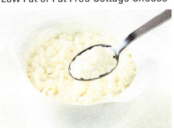

Tofu

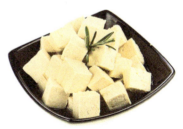

Healthy Fats: Monounsaturated & Omega-3 Polyunsaturated Fatty Acids:
Extra virgin olive oil, nuts, avocados, seeds, soy foods

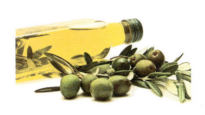

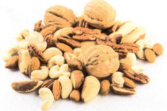

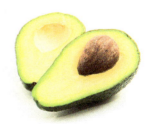

Figure 3
All images © Shutterstock, Inc.

Anti-Inflammatory Drinks

Green Tea

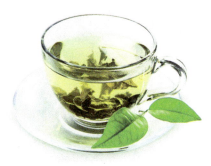

Soy Milk

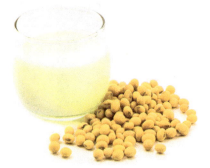

Water

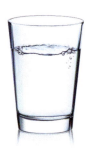

Tart Cherry Juice

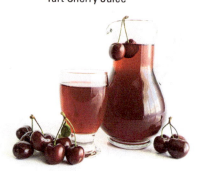

Fresh Fruit & Vegetable Smoothies & Juices

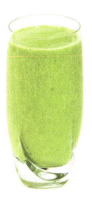
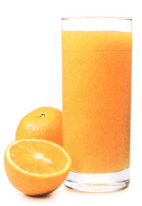

Figure 4
All images © Shutterstock, Inc.

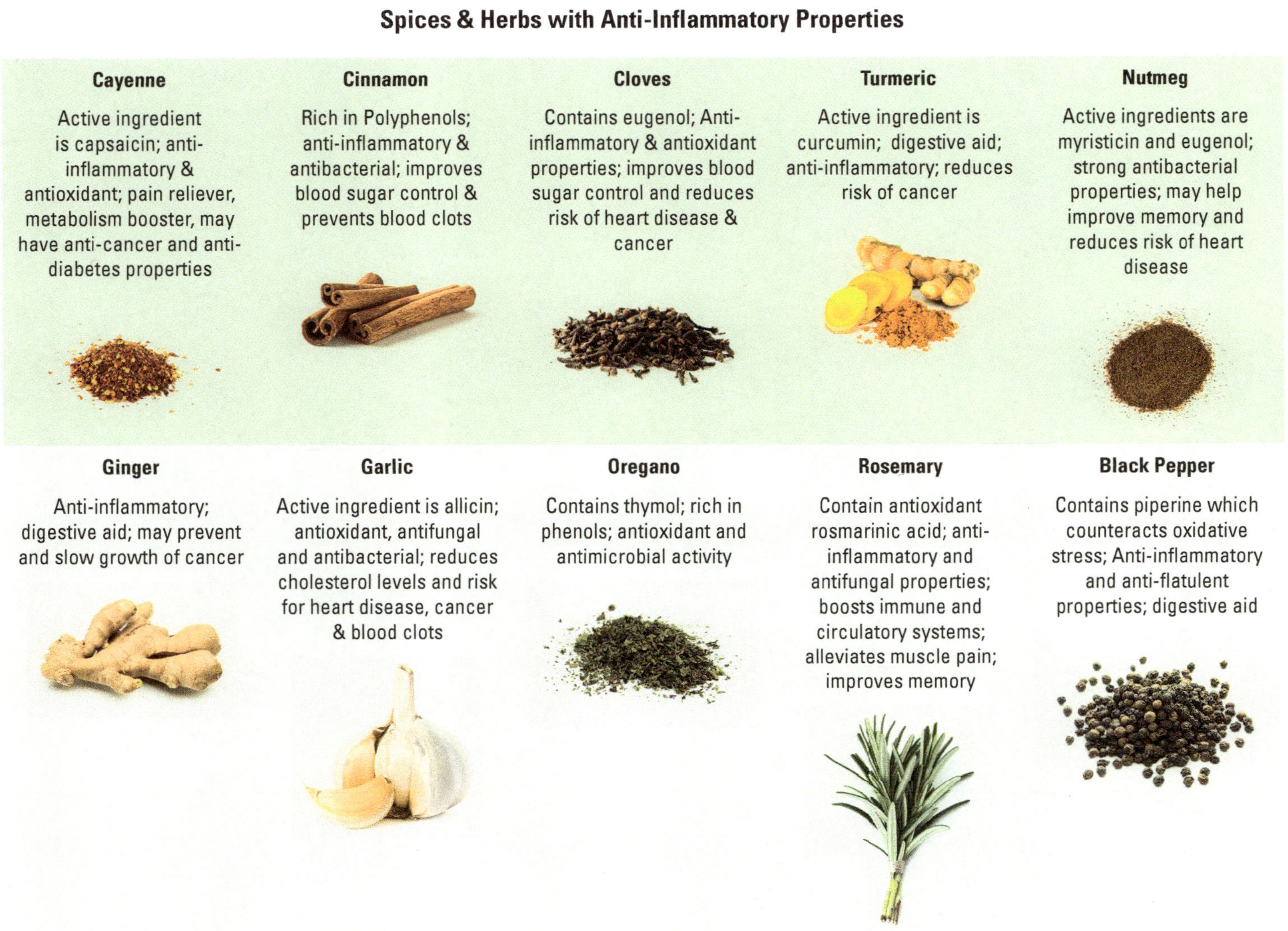

Nutrition & Your Health 45

Spices & Herbs with Anti-Inflammatory Properties

Cayenne
Active ingredient is capsaicin; anti-inflammatory & antioxidant; pain reliever, metabolism booster, may have anti-cancer and anti-diabetes properties

Cinnamon
Rich in Polyphenols; anti-inflammatory & antibacterial; improves blood sugar control & prevents blood clots

Cloves
Contains eugenol; Anti-inflammatory & antioxidant properties; improves blood sugar control and reduces risk of heart disease & cancer

Turmeric
Active ingredient is curcumin; digestive aid; anti-inflammatory; reduces risk of cancer

Nutmeg
Active ingredients are myristicin and eugenol; strong antibacterial properties; may help improve memory and reduces risk of heart disease

Ginger
Anti-inflammatory; digestive aid; may prevent and slow growth of cancer

Garlic
Active ingredient is allicin; antioxidant, antifungal and antibacterial; reduces cholesterol levels and risk for heart disease, cancer & blood clots

Oregano
Contains thymol; rich in phenols; antioxidant and antimicrobial activity

Rosemary
Contain antioxidant rosmarinic acid; anti-inflammatory and antifungal properties; boosts immune and circulatory systems; alleviates muscle pain; improves memory

Black Pepper
Contains piperine which counteracts oxidative stress; Anti-inflammatory and anti-flatulent properties; digestive aid

Figure 5
All images © Shutterstock, Inc.

Positive Mental Health
Flow & Flourishing

"The best moments in our lives are not the passive, receptive, relaxing times . . . The best moments usually occur if a person's body or mind is stretched to its limits in a voluntary effort to accomplish something difficult and worthwhile."

—Mihaly Csikszentmihalyi

Overview

So far in this semester, class content has touched on many physical aspects of health, including stress, sleep, physical activity, and nutrition. This week's focus is on mental and emotional health.

In the 1990s, a scientific and professional movement in psychology began seeking to better understand what is "right" or "good" with people. The goal of this movement is to better understand and build the enabling conditions that make life worth living. Dr. Martin Seligman was integral in the movement by bringing together and moving forward the scientific inquiry of what is now called "positive psychology." Positive psychology has been conceptualized as the scientific study of human strengths and virtues that contribute to optimal functioning and flourishing. It is important to note that positive psychology is not intended to replace therapy or pharmacology.

Happiness, flow, meaning, love, gratitude, accomplishment, growth, and better relationships are all pieces of the puzzle that constitutes human flourishing. Research done by Dr. Corey Keyes indicates that any state of mental health that is less than flourishing imposes a burden on the individual and society. As only a small percentage of people who are free from mental illness are actually "flourishing," the need to enhance positive mental states is clear (Keyes, 2007).

One of the elements of flourishing and happiness is "flow." Hungarian psychologist Csikszentmihalyi (1990), one of the founders of positive psychology and who did the pioneering research on flow, defined "flow" as a state in which people become completely immersed in an activity where their level of skill matches the challenge at hand. In his book *Flow—The Psychology of Optimal Experience*, he describes certain characteristics of flow activities. These include clear goals, immediate feedback, intrinsic reward, concentration, merging of action and awareness, transformation of time, feeling in control, and balance between skills and challenges.

Interestingly, research in the field of positive psychology seems to indicate that positive states not only affect mental and emotional health, but physical health as well. In his book *Flourish*, Dr. Seligman illustrates how optimism and positive emotion may be associated with protection from physical ailments, such as cardiovascular disease, colds and flu, and possibly cancer (Seligman, 2011).

This week in class you will explore positive mental health concepts and have the opportunity to cultivate flow experiences by incorporating them into your personal health goal and action steps.

Learning Objectives

1. Identify the key components of Positive Psychology.
2. Compare and contrast the traditional versus positive psychology approach to the health–disease continuum.
3. Describe two ways in which having a positive outlook affects health.
4. Explain how engaging in flow activities contributes to health.
5. Analyze how engaging in flow activities encourages academic success.
6. Evaluate your activities for flow experiences.
7. Integrate flow activities into the action steps for your health goal.

Knowledge Nuggets

Flow is unique for each person depending on skill level, interest, and other personal characteristics. An activity that gets one person "in the flow zone" may induce boredom or anxiety in another (Rogatko, 2009).

A popular metaphor for describing the difference between positive psychology and traditional psychology is that while the general work of psychology can be seen as learning how to bring people up from negative eight to zero, positive psychology attempts to understand how to bring people up from zero to positive eight (Gable & Haidt, 2005).

People's level of positivity in the present provides a happiness advantage to the brain. Your brain at positive is 31% more productive than your brain at negative, neutral, or stressed (Achor, 2011).

Positive Mental Health: Flow & Flourishing

☑ Pre-Work

- ❏ Watch: Online Presentation—Flow & Flourishing.
- ❏ Read: Chapters 1 and 2 of *Flourish* by Martin E.P. Seligman.
- ❏ Watch video: Shawn Achor TED Talk, "The Happiness Advantage: Linking Positive Brains to Performance."

✎ In-Class Activity: Flow and Tell

In a small group, generate a list of several activities that you typically engage in as well as activities that you are passionate about making time to do. List at least five in the space below.

Considering your experience during these activities, determine if they meet the flow criteria (clear goals, immediate feedback, intrinsic reward, concentration, merging of action and awareness, transformation of time, feeling in control, and balance between skills and challenges). If the activity meets few of the criteria, it is likely a low flow experience. If the activity meets several of the criteria, it is likely a high flow activity.

Activity	Level of Flow?
1. Fencing	**High** or Low
2. Studying	High or **Low**
3. Running	**High** or Low
4. _____	High or Low
5. _____	High or Low

As a group, discuss the following questions. Be prepared to share the answers with the class.

1. Which activities met more conditions for flow?

2. Were any activities considered high flow by some in the group and low flow by others? Why might this be the case?

3. Consider the values and character strengths content from a few weeks ago. What values or strengths are in play when you are engaging in an activity that induces flow?

4. How can character strengths be utilized to cultivate more flow when engaging in a low flow activity?

   For example: Susie finds that course work in a required class does not particularly interest her. Her top three character strengths are social intelligence, self-regulation, and creativity. Because of her self-regulation, she decides to make a study schedule while using her social intelligence and creativity to organize a study group. Together, the group was able to make the course material more interesting by sharing their perspectives and understanding of the material.

5. How can you create opportunities to experience flow more regularly?

☑ Post-Work

- ❏ Assignment: Complete Goal Worksheet #3 and submit online.

🛠 Additional Tips and Resources

- Count your blessings.

  Consider completing the Three Blessings exercise mentioned in Seligman's Flourish. For one week, every night before you go to sleep, write down three good things that happened that day. Then reflect on why they happened. This practice helps you to focus and acknowledge the positive things that happen in your life.

- Be grateful.

  Practicing gratitude has linked to more optimistic life appraisals, more time exercising, and improved well-being (Emmons & McCullough, 2003). Take time every day to notice when someone does something nice for you (or others). Actively acknowledge and thank them! It's a simple and easy way to express gratitude.

- Interested in learning more about flow and peak performance?

  Check out Mihaly Csikszentmihalyi's groundbreaking classic book *Flow: The Psychology of Optimal Experience*.

❓ Study Questions

What is positive psychology?

What are the five elements of Seligman's Well-Being Theory?

What is positive affect?

What is flourishing? What is the opposite of flourishing?

What is the difference between mental health and mental illness?

What is the relevance of flourishing in college students? How does it relate to academic success?

List some evidence-based tips for increasing positive affect and flourishing

List the seven elements of flow.

Be familiar with the skills and challenge chart for flow.

    Where must challenge and skill level be to be in a state of flow?

    What is it called when you have a high challenge level and a low skill level?

    What is it called when you have a moderate skill level but a low challenge level?

What is the relationship between flow and academics?

How does positive affect protect against inflammatory disorders?

What body systems does flow affect? What are the effects of this?

What elements of happiness are associated with flow?

Sleep & Your Health

"Sleep is the golden chain that ties health and our bodies together."
—Thomas Dekker

🏛 Overview

Did you know that we spend one-third of our lives asleep? What purpose might these periods of reduced alertness serve? As sleep is often an underappreciated component of success and well-being in college, it is the goal of this module to examine the many benefits of sleep and understand why we should prioritize our rest.

Why do we need sleep? Sleep plays a vital role in memory consolidation for motor skills (Walker et al., 2002a), visual tasks (Karni et al., 1994), auditory skills (Gaab et al., 2004), and fact-based memory (De Koninck et al., 1989). Problem solving (Walker et al., 2002b) and insight (Wagner et al., 2004) improve with sleep. Sleep may eliminate toxic proteins that build up while we are awake (Xie et al., 2013). Hence, a lack of sleep produces a range of deleterious effects.

An abundance of evidence demonstrates that sleep promotes optimal physical health. Long-term consequences of compromised sleep include an increased risk of cancer, cardiovascular disease, type II diabetes, and obesity (Luyster et al., 2012). Significant physical changes, however, also occur in the short term. When individuals sleep for only four hours per night for two consecutive nights, appetite increases and blood sugar level regulation is perturbed (Spiegel et al., 2004, 2005). A single night of sleep deprivation can alter immune response up to four weeks later, and

> Chronic inflammation can be triggered by long-term shortened sleep cycles. When sleep is interrupted or you sleep too few hours, you do not get enough Delta phase sleep. Delta is the phase of sleep where tissue micro-trauma is repaired. Inadequate repair results in low level tissue trauma, which can produce sustained, generalized inflammation.

an average sleep duration of less than seven hours per night for two weeks increases susceptibility to the common cold (Cohen et al., 2009; Lange et al., 2003).

Do you feel irritable when you don't sleep enough? Reduced sleep impairs emotional regulation, often leading to increased anger, irritability, and confusion (Baum et al., 2014), resulting in heightened emotional responses, sensitivity to stress (Minkel et al., 2012), decreased empathy (Guadagni et al., 2014), and diminished trust (Anderson & Dickinson, 2010). Sleep disturbances may precede the onset of depression and other mood disorders (Ohayon & Roth, 2003).

Do you feel fuzzy-headed when you don't sleep? Lack of sufficient sleep is associated with an increase in human error-related accidents (Dinges, 1995) and increased impulsivity (Anderson & Platten, 2011). One or two nights of total sleep deprivation, or 2 weeks of less than 6 hours per night, impairs cognitive processing speed, working memory, and attention (Van Dongen et al., 2003). Effects of chronic sleep insufficiency extend to memory loss (Scullin & Bliwise, 2015) and increased risk for neurological disorders (Palma, Urrestarazu, & Iriarte, 2013).

The National Sleep Foundation recommends that young adults (aged 18–25 years old) get seven to nine hours of sleep each night (Hirshkowitz et al., 2015). Most college students, however, do not meet this recommendation (Hershner & Chervin, 2014; Lund et al., 2010). This module aims to demonstrate the importance of sleep to your health and the value of developing effective time management strategies to achieve a balance between schoolwork, extracurricular activities, and social events.

Learning Objectives

1. Identify common factors that lead to insufficient sleep for college students.
2. Discuss the evidence that sleep deprivation has negative consequences for:
    a. physical health;
    b. mental health; and
    c. cognitive performance.
3. Examine the benefits of sleep that are applicable to college students on a daily basis.
4. Describe potential strategies to improve sleep.

Knowledge Nuggets

Inadequate sleep is correlated with multiple physical and mental health issues, including cardiovascular disease, diabetes, obesity, neurodegenerative disorders, depression, and anxiety. Experimental studies have demonstrated that sleep disruption lasting only a day or two is sufficient to alter many biological processes.

Lack of sufficient sleep has negative consequences for cognitive functioning, including attention, memory, and reaction time. The deficits observed after sleep deprivation are similar to those caused by alcohol. Experimentally, a single night of sleep deprivation has been shown to demonstrate the same decline in cognitive performance as seen in someone with a blood alcohol level of 0.1 (percent by volume), which is above the legal limit to drive in the United States.

Barriers to sleep in college students include inadequate sleep time, erratic sleep schedules, sleep disorders, caffeine and energy drinks, technology, excess noise, and stress. Maximize sleep quality by optimizing your sleep habits and sleep environment.

Student Story

Natalie was having trouble focusing and staying awake in class. She usually finished her day and got into bed around 10:00 p.m. every night but didn't fall asleep right away. Even though she was in bed early, Natalie often ended up doing last minute work or watching Netflix before trying to sleep. During this time, she got hungry and would grab snacks from her bedside table and eat them in bed. Because of this, she found herself wired at night and wouldn't become tired until a few hours after she got into bed, so she only received about 5 hours of sleep each day.

Natalie tried going to bed earlier but it didn't help. She then decided to start finishing her homework at her desk before getting into bed and switched to reading a book for 30 minutes rather than watching Netflix. She made sure to keep food stored away from her bedside table. She found this helpful because she started to associate her bed with sleep. Now, every time she gets into bed, she is able to relax and is more readily able to fall asleep.

Pre-Work

- ❏ Watch: Online Presentation.
- ❏ Read: Chapter 7 of *Sleep: A Very Short Introduction* by Steven W. Lockley and Russell G. Foster.
- ❏ Assignment: Complete sleep log (start 7 days prior to due date) and submit online. Bring a copy with you to class.

In-Class Activity

Sleep disturbances and sleep deprivation are very common issues for college students. This activity will help identify the most common barriers to getting sufficient sleep and strategies for addressing them.

Discussion questions

- What was the average amount of sleep per night across the class?

- The study by Lund et al. (2010), which was discussed in the online presentation, found that only half of college students reported meeting the recommended minimum of 7 hours of sleep per night. How does this class compare?

- How much did the average amount of sleep differ between weeknights and weekends? What factors contribute to this difference?

- Were there differences in how rested individuals felt, or in other words in how they experienced daytime sleepiness during the week versus weekends?

- What were the most common factors that caused a delay from when you intended to go to sleep?

- What were the most common factors that disrupted sleep in the middle of the night? Do certain dorms have more of an issue with noise than others?

- How has your sleep changed since coming to college? Do you get more or less sleep than you did during high school? Explain any different factors that disrupt your sleep in college.

- What strategies have you tried to address your sleep difficulties? What factors that cause sleep disruption do you still need to address?

- Take a couple of minutes to draw a picture of your ideal sleep environment. How did the characteristics of these environments compare across the class? What factors did you include that were included in the tips discussed in the online presentation? What could you do to increase the potential for better quality sleep in this environment?

☑ Post-Work: None

✗ Additional Tips and Resources

- Set your alarm—to go to bed.

  If you consistently find yourself wishing you could get more sleep and struggle with a calming bedtime routine, program a reminder or signal as a cue that it's time to wind up things for the day and go to bed.

- Keep your bedroom like a cave—dark, cool, and quiet.

  The glow from a digital clock, noise, and being too warm can keep you from going and staying asleep. Consider using an eye mask, ear plugs and aim for a room temperature in the mid-60 degree Fahrenheit range.

- Wondering how good your sleep really is?

  Using a phone app like *Sleep Time* gives you insight into the duration and efficiency of your sleep.

❓ Study Questions

What deficits are associated with a lack of sleep? How prevalent are these deficits? How much sleep loss must occur to observe these deficits?

What diseases or disorders are commonly associated with sleep complaints?

What factors commonly cause sleep disruptions? Are these disruptive factors linked with any other health issues?

How prominent are sleep difficulties in college students? What are the negative consequences of insufficient sleep that negatively affect academic performance?

What two processes regulate sleep quantity and timing?

What relationships or associations exist between sleep disturbances and mental health?

How is mortality related to sleep duration?

What physical health outcomes are associated with short sleep duration? What evidence exists to support these links?

What mental health outcomes are associated with short sleep duration? What evidence exists to support these links?

What cognitive impairments are associated with short sleep duration? What evidence exists to support these links?

Consider the physical health outcomes, mental health outcomes, and cognitive impairments associated with short sleep duration. Explain the relevance of these outcomes in the daily life of a college student.

What is the recommended amount of sleep for young adults?

What insufficient sleep-related complaints are frequently reported by college students?

How can you make your sleeping environment more conducive to better quality sleep?

Physical Activity & Your Health

"The mechanisms by which exercise changes how we think and feel are so much more effective than donuts, medicines, and wine. At every level, from the microcellular to the psychological, exercise not only wards off the ill effects of chronic stress; it can also reverse them."

—John Ratey, author of Spark

Overview

Academic success is a priority in college, and it's often tempting to push aside exercise in favor of hitting the books. A recent report showed that only approximately 42% of undergraduate students were meeting the public health guidelines for moderate-vigorous physical activity per week. Yet contrary to common belief, the students who were meeting the exercise recommendations were found to have a higher grade point average than those who were not (Keating, Castelli, & Ayers, 2013; Wald, 2014). In what other ways could exercise improve your college experience? There are many well-known health benefits of regular physical activity, from improved body composition to reduced risk of chronic illness and premature death (US Department of Health and Human Services, 2008). But exercise provides so many more benefits: it helps us think more clearly and feel happier. These effects on our cognitive and emotional health are less commonly appreciated. It is the goal of this module to specifically explore these areas and expand your understanding of how exercise has an impact on all pillars of health.

Everyone knows that exercise is a good thing to do, but how much is required to reap the rewards? Engaging in at least 150 minutes per week of moderate-vigorous physical activity or at least 75 minutes of vigorous activity is recommended to gain most of the health benefits of exercise. Meeting these guidelines reduces an individual's risk for developing many chronic diseases and dying prematurely. It also helps with prevention of weight gain and results in improved cardiorespiratory and muscular fitness. Even more health benefits are gained with more time spent in aerobic activity, as well as if a person engages in muscle-strengthening activities at least two or more days per week (US Department of Health and Human Services, 2008). In fact, having a high level of cardiorespiratory fitness is one of the most powerful ways to prevent chronic disease. Participating in various activities that you enjoy can help you reach this goal!

Did you know that some of these health outcomes are also improved by reducing the amount of time you are sedentary? Sedentary behaviors are activities that involve sitting, reclining, or laying down during waking hours (Matthews, 2008). It is estimated that American adults spend at least 60% of daily waking hours sedentary in activities such as using the computer, watching television, or commuting in an automobile—that's a minimum of about 8 hours per day! Spending more time in sedentary behaviors increases a person's risk of dying prematurely and developing many chronic diseases—even if he or she meets the weekly recommendations for exercise. However, the good news is that replacing sedentary behaviors with light activities that require standing and slow walking helps reduce the risk of adverse health outcomes (Dempsey, 2014; Katzmarzyk, 2009; Owen, 2010).

A *neat* way to think about this is that replacing sitting with light intensity activities increases non-exercise activity thermogenesis (NEAT). NEAT is the amount of energy expended by the body to carry out all activities that are not sleeping, eating, or sports-like exercise. For example, an office worker who wants to increase his NEAT could conduct some meetings while walking, park further away from the office building or commute to work by bike, take a walk at lunch, or convert to a standing desk; these changes could increase NEAT by up to 10-fold, or approximately 500–1,000 kcal per day (Levine, 2015). Other studies show that splitting up sitting time into shorter chunks with more frequent breaks also improves disease biomarkers compared to sitting for the same amount of time with less frequent breaks. One study showed that compared to frequent breakers, prolonged sitters had increased waist circumference, body mass index, plasma triglycerides, and two-hour blood glucose levels, which are risk factors for type 2 diabetes and cardiovascular disease (Owen, 2010). For your health, try not to sit, and if you must sit, move often—and stay fit!

One way to estimate whether you are moving enough is to track how many steps you take each day. Scientists who study sedentary behavior have proposed recommendations for how many steps per day are enough and how many are too few, according to the following categories: *Sedentary* = less than 5,000 steps/day; *Low Active* = 5,000–7,499 steps/day; *Somewhat Active* = 7,500–9,999 steps/day; *Active* = 10,000–12,499 steps/day; and *Highly Active* = greater than or equal to 12,500 steps/day (Tudor-Locke et al., 2008). Accumulating less than 5,000 steps/day is consistently associated with less favorable body composition and markers of cardiovascular disease risk. Young adults who decreased steps from over 10,000 to less than 5,000/day experienced increased adiposity, decreased insulin sensitivity and glucose control, and other unfavorable health changes within three to fourteen days of reduced activity levels (Tudor-Locke et al., 2011). The tiered steps per day recommendations reflect that any exercise is better than none, and more health benefits are seen with more movement. Therefore, to be *active*, an adult should aim to accumulate at least 10,000 steps/, and even more if possible.

Getting up and moving not only helps prevent disease, but it also makes you feel and think better. Cognitive function and exercise work hand-in-hand. While the brain regulates our ability to move, exercise has direct effects on brain functions (Loprenzi et al., 2013). Exercise has been found to alter the structure and function of multiple brain areas that result in enhanced cognitive functions, including increased mental flexibility, concentration skills, and memory (Bucci & Hopkins, 2010; Themanson, Pontifex, & Hillman, 2008; van Praag et al., 2014). These cognitive improvements can be partially attributed to increased levels of a specific chemical, brain-derived neurotropic factor (BDNF), which is fundamental to the health of brain cells. BDNF enhances the survival and function of neurons, and improves their resistance to damage from oxidative and metabolic stress (Mattson, 2012; van Praag et al., 2014). Increased neuronal formation and cellular stress reduction improve your mental functioning in the near term and stave off depression and the negative effects of aging associated with a decline in neuron formation (van Praag et al., 2014).

Beyond altering the inner workings of our brains, exercise has direct effects on our emotional health. Mood in general and specific symptoms of mood-related disorders have been demonstrated to be highly influenced by physical activity (Herring et al., 2011; van Praag et al., 2014). For example, among women with generalized anxiety disorder, six weeks of resistance and/or aerobic exercise training resulted in noticeably improved levels of irritability, anxiety, vigor, and pain (Herring et al, 2011). Moreover, active individuals have been found to report symptoms of depression 45% less frequently than inactive individuals (Physical Activity Guidelines Advisory Committee, 2008). Impressively, vigorously active college students report lower anxiety and fewer depressive symptoms than those with low activity levels (Brand et al., 2010). Possible mechanisms underlying these relationships are skeletal muscle changes that mediate resilience to inflammation and stress-induced depression (Agudelo et al., 2014) and/or improved sleep quality (Brand et al., 2010). As depression and anxiety have been reported to affect approximately one in five undergraduate students, and poor psychological health negatively impacts academic performance, exercise is a fundamental strategy for maintaining sound mental and emotional health in college (Ruthig et al., 2011).

The demands of college life can often be overwhelming, causing your physical, mental, and emotional health to suffer. By the end of the module, you should consider how sitting less and setting aside time to regularly participate in physical activity is a good strategy to combat stress, achieve your goals, and work toward being the best version of yourself.

Learning Objectives

1. Summarize how exercise is beneficial to your health.
2. Explain the effects of exercise on the brain and the related associations with academic performance.
3. Compare and contrast how ghrelin and leptin effect appetite and explain how these are modified by exercise.

4. Describe the relationship between exercise and sleep.

5. Consider the importance of exercise for immune health and outline specific benefits toward decreased inflammation.

Knowledge Nuggets

Regular exercise is associated with improved cognition, memory, and sleep quality (Brand et al., 2010; Bucci & Hopkins, 2010; van Praag et al., 2014).

Exercise is an effective method to improve mood through alleviation of anxiety and depression (Agudelo et al., 2014; Herring et al, 2011).

Moving our muscles produces proteins that travel through the bloodstream and into the brain, where they play pivotal roles in the mechanisms of our highest thought processes (Ratey & Hagerman, 2008).

Student Story

Back in high school, Laura was in the habit of exercising daily for an hour at the gym. However, after coming to college, she found herself more pressed for time and only worked out once every two weeks. She didn't feel motivated to work out on the machines in WoodPec, because she found it boring. Plus, she would rather stay in bed after a day of school, because she had no energy. Laura had gotten sick twice so far in the semester, felt groggy all the time, and was often stress eating.

Laura decided that since she realized she had no motivation to go to the gym after school, she got up early every morning to work out. This helped her sleep, since she had a more structured schedule, and her stress eating had been significantly reduced. Since the WoodPec workout area didn't help motivate her to exercise, she decided to buy an unlimited Class Card for the Fitness Classes instead. She took various classes, including Yoga, Zumba, and Spinning. If it was nice outside, she went for a run or walk around Lullwater because it gave her a chance to leave campus. With these changes, she began to notice she got sick much less often, was less stressed, and happier overall.

Pre-Work

- ❏ Watch: Online Presentation—Exercise.
- ❏ Read: *Spark: The Revolutionary New Science of Exercise and the Brain* (Ratey), Introduction and Chapters 1 and 10.
- ❏ Assignment: Complete the physical activity log in your workbook (start seven days prior to due date) and take a picture to submit online. Bring your workbook to class.

Instructions for completing the assignment:

1. Track your daily steps.

   Use a pedometer to track the number of steps you take each day. You can do this with an app for your mobile phone or a traditional clip-on pedometer.

   There are many free phone apps for iPhone and Android that have pedometer functions. Some newer phones come with apps already installed, so check your phone to see if you need to install one or not. **Argus** and **Pacer** are two examples that are free and available for both iPhone and Android.

   If you prefer to use a traditional clip-on pedometer, a limited number are available for loan from the CSHH main office in Candler Library Room 107.

2. Fill out the physical activity log. Each day, write down your activities in the appropriate boxes, and add up approximately how much time (hours, minutes) you participated in each type of activity.

   - Sedentary activities involve sitting or reclining.
   - Exercise activities occur for at least ten minutes at a time. They increase your heart rate and cause you to breathe harder. Some examples of exercise include brisk walking, jogging or running, lifting weights, using cardio equipment at the gym, doing Yoga, playing sports, etc.
   - Each night before you go to bed, look at your pedometer information and write down how many steps you took throughout the day.
   - Note how many hours you were awake each day.
   - In the comments box, write down anything else notable about the day. (For example: Were you stressed out due to a big exam? Did you have a fantastic day and meet all your goals? Were you overly tired or extra-energized? Did something unexpected happen that kept you from meeting your daily goals?)

3. Take a picture of your physical activity log after *writing your name and section number* in the spaces provided and upload it to Blackboard before your HLTH 100 class. Bring your workbook to class.

Physical Activity & Your Health

Name: Christopher Dong
HLTH 100 section: 055

	Sedentary Activities (type, duration)	Exercises (type, duration)	Steps Taken per Day	Awake Time	Comments
Day 1	Studying Gaming Lazing about Eating 14:00 — Total time	Fencing 1:00 — Total time	3358	16:00	Lots work and little time to move about
Day 2	Studying Gaming Lazing about Eating 13:38 — Total time	Jogging Fencing 2:00 — Total time	5215	16:38	Plenty of bladework without foot movement
Day 3	Studying Eating 10:52 — Total time	N/A 0:00 — Total time	1538	12:24	Slept quite a bit. Worked a lot.
Day 4	Studying Eating 9:43 — Total time	Fencing 0:30 — Total time	1692	11:18	More studying and sleeping
Day 5	Studying Gaming Lazing about Eating 12:50 — Total time	Fencing 2:00 — Total time	7386	15:48	Lots fencing work.
Day 6	Studying Gaming Lazing about Eating 13:00 — Total time	Fencing 1:00 — Total time	4918	15:00	Fencing was mixed.
Average	12:21	1:05	4018	14:31	An ok week

In-Class Activity: Physical Activity Log Discussion

- Use your average values from your completed physical activity log and calculate the percentage of awake time you spent in sedentary behaviors and in exercise for the week.

- What was the average amount of awake time, sedentary time, exercise time, and steps/day for the class?

- A 2014 study by Wald et al. found that only about 42% of college students meet public health recommendations for cardiovascular and muscle-strengthening exercise each week. How does this class compare?

- What were sedentary behaviors common to class members?

- Have your patterns of exercise or sedentary behaviors changed since coming to college? How and why?

- Consider the average number of steps taken per day for the whole class. Under what steps per day category does the class fall?

- How did your movement patterns relate to how you felt each day? Did you notice whether sitting a lot, moving around a lot, and/or participating in exercise impacted how you thought, felt, or functioned?

- Do you want to change anything about your usual movement patterns? What are specific strategies you can use?

- Do you anticipate any barriers to changing your movement patterns? What are potential solutions?

- Can changing your movement patterns support your health goal that you have been updating throughout the semester? If so, how? If not, why not?

- How can you use movement/exercise to improve all of your pillars of health?

☑ Post-Work: None

🛠 Additional Tips and Resources

- Increase your NEAT

    Get creative around campus by taking a longer route between classes, using the stairs to get to your classroom, and standing up while hanging out and talking to friends in the dorm. When studying, set a reminder on your computer or phone that signals you to get up and move around every hour. Use this opportunity to get some water, go outside for some fresh air, or stretch your arms and legs.

- Find an exercise buddy

    Be social and physically active by working out with a friend. Having a partner to exercise with can help you stay motivated and on track with your activity goals. A good workout buddy provides support and accountability in a positive and encouraging way.

- American College of Sports Medicine http://www.acsm.org/public-information.

- Emory Recreation and Wellness: Facilities, Fitness, Intramurals, Club Sports, etc. http://www.play.emory.edu/.

❓ Study Questions

How do physical fitness and sedentary behaviors relate to health outcomes?

How does exercise training affect the brain?

What protein is responsible for cognitive improvements associated with exercise?

What part of the brain shows functional improvements in memory retention with aerobic exercise?

In general, how does exercise affect memory?

How does exercise influence psychological well-being?

What are specific effects of exercise on sleep?

By what hormonal mechanisms does exercise influence appetite?

What is the relationship between exercise and immunity?

How is exercise anti-inflammatory?

References

Achor, S. "The Happy Secret to Better Work." *TEDxBloomington* 2011. Web. 15 June 2015.

Agudelo, LZ, et al. "Skeletal Muscle PGC-1α1 Modulates Kynurenine Metabolism and Mediates Resilience to Stress-Induced Depression." *Cell* 159.1 (2014): 33–45.

American College Health Association-National College Health Assessment II: Institutional Data Report Fall 2011 Emory University. Hanover, MD: American College Health Association; 2011. Customized analysis provided by Marc Cordon, MPH and Kirsten Bondalapati.

Anderson, C, and Dickinson, DL. "Bargaining and Trust: The Effects of 36-h Total Sleep Deprivation on Socially Interactive Decisions." *Journal of Sleep Research* 19 (2010): 54–63.

Anderson, C, and Platten, CR. "Sleep Deprivation Lowers Inhibition and Enhances Impulsivity to Negative Stimuli." *Behavioral Brain Research* 217 (2011): 463–466.

Baum, KT, et al. "Sleep Restriction Worsens Mood and Emotion Regulation in Adolescents." *Journal of Child Psychology and Psychiatry, and Allied Disciplines* 55 (2014): 180–190.

Brand, S, et al. "High Exercise Levels Are Related to Favorable Sleep Patterns and Psychological Functioning in Adolescents: A Comparison of Athletes and Controls." *Journal of Adolescent Health* 46.2 (2010): 133–141.

Brunner, EJ, et al. "Dietary Patterns and 15-Y Risks of Major Coronary Events, Diabetes, and Mortality." *The American Journal of Clinical Nutrition* 87.5 (2008): 1414–1421.

BRFSS 2011 Survey Data and Documentation: http://www.cdc.gov/brfss/annual_data/annual_2011.htm.

Bucci, DJ, and Hopkins, ME. "BDNF Expression in Peripheral Cortex is Associated with Exercise-Induced Improvement in Object Recognition Memory." *Neurobiology of Learning and Memory* 94.2 (2010): 278–284.

Bull, Fiona C, Kreuter, Matthew W, and Scharff, Darcell P. "Effects of Tailored, Personalized and General Health Messages on Physical Activity." *Patient Education and Counseling* 36.2 (1999): 181–192. Web.

Campbell, RL, Svenson, LW, and Jarvis, GK. "Perceived Level of Stress among University Undergraduate Students in Edmonton, Canada." *Perceptual and Motor Skills* 75 (1992): 552–554.

Corporate Leadership Council. "2002 Performance Management Survey. Formal Performance Review." *Building the High-Performance Workforce*. Washington, DC: Corporate Leadership Council, 2002, p. 29a.

Cohen, S, et al. "Sleep Habits and Susceptibility to the Common Cold." *Archives of Internal Medicine* 169 (2009): 62–67.

Creswell, J, et al. "Affirmation of Personal Values Buffers Neuroendocrine and Psychological Response to Stress." *Psychological Science* 16.11 (2005): 846–851.

Csikszentmihalyi, M. *Flow: The Psychology of Optimal Experience*. New York, NY: Harper and Row, 1990. Print.

De Koninck, J, et al. "Intensive Language Learning and Increases in Rapid Eye Movement Sleep: Evidence of a Performance Factor." *International Journal of Psychophysiology* 8 (1989): 43–47.

Dempsey PC, Owen N, Biddle SJ, Dunstan DW. "Managing sedentary behavior to reduce the risk of diabetes and cardiovascular disease." *Curr Diab Rep.* 2014;14(9):522. doi: 10.1007/s11892-014-0522-0. Web.

de Vries, H, et al. "The Effectiveness of Tailored Feedback and Action Plans in an Intervention Addressing Multiple Health Behaviors." *American Journal of Health Promotion* 22.6 (2008): 417–425.

Dinges, DF. "An Overview of Sleepiness and Accidents." *Journal of Sleep Research* 4 (1995): 4–14.

Doran, George T. "There's a S.M.A.R.T. Way to Write Management's Goals and Objectives." *Management Review* 70.11 (1981): 35–36.

Emmons, RA, and McCullough, ME. "Counting Blessings Versus Burdens: An Experimental Investigation of Gratitude and Subjective Well-Being in Daily Life." *Journal of Personality and Social Psychology* 84 (2003): 377–389.

Friedlander, Laura J, et al. "Social Support, Self-Esteem, and Stress as Predictors of Adjustment to University among First-Year Undergraduates." *Journal of College Student Development* 48.3 (2007): 259–274.

Gaab, N, et al. "The Influence of Sleep on Auditory Learning: A Behavioral Study." *Neuroreport* 15.4 (2004): 731–734.

Gable, Shelly L, and Haidt, Jonathan. "What (And Why) Is Positive Psychology?" *Review of General Psychology* 9.2 (2005): 103–110. Web.

Gazzara, Kevin. "SMART Goals History with Dr. George Doran." Online video clip. *YouTube.* Web. https://youtu.be/7LWbCqjLE-I. 12 September 2010.

Govindji, Reena, and Linley, Alex P. "Strengths Use, Self-concordance and Well-being: Implications for Strengths Coaching and Coaching Psychologists." *International Coaching Psychology Review* 2.2 (2007): 143–153.

Guadagni, V, et al. "The Effects of Sleep Deprivation on Emotional Empathy. *Journal of Sleep Research* 23 (2014): 657–663.

Herring, MP, et al. "Effects of Short-Term Exercise Training on Signs and Symptoms of GAD." *Mental Health and Physical Activity* 4 (2011): 71–77.

Hershner, SD, and Chervin, RD. "Causes and Consequences of Sleepiness among College Students." *Nature and Science of Sleep* 6 (2014): 73–84.

Hirshkowitz, M, et al. "National Sleep Foundation's Sleep Time Duration Recommendations: Methodology and Results Summary." *Sleep Health* 1 (2015): 40–43.

Howitz, KT, and Sinclair, DA. "Xenohormesis: Sensing the Chemical Cues of Other Species." *Cell* 133 (2008): 387–391.

Institute of Medicine (US) Committee on Sleep Medicine and Research; Colten HR, Altevogt BM, editors. *Sleep Disorders and Sleep Deprivation: An Unmet Public Health Problem.* Washington (DC): National Academies Press (US); 2006. "3, Extent and Health Consequences of Chronic Sleep Loss and Sleep Disorders." Available from: http://www.ncbi.nlm.nih.gov/books/NBK19961/.

Kadison, Richard, and DiGeronimo, Theresa Foy. *College of the Overwhelmed: The Campus Mental Health Crisis and What to Do About It.* San Francisco, CA: Jossey-Bass, 2004.

Karni, A, et al. "Dependence on REM Sleep of Overnight Improvement of a Perceptual Skill." *Science* 265 (1994): 679–682.

Katzmarzyk, PT, et al. "Sitting Time and Mortality from All Causes, Cardiovascular Disease, and Cancer." *Medicine and Science in Sports and Exercise* 41.5 (2009): 998–1005.

Keating, XD, Castelli, D, and Ayers, SF. "Association of Weekly Strength Exercise Frequency and Academic Performance among Students at a Large University in the United States." *Journal of Strength and Conditioning Research* 27.7 (2013): 1988–1993.

Keyes, CL. "Promoting and Protecting Mental Health as Flourishing: A Complementary Strategy for Improving National Mental Health." *American Psychologist* 62.2 (2007): 95–108.

Kiecolt-Glaser, Janice K. "Stress, Food, and Inflammation: Psychoneuroimmunology and Nutrition at the Cutting Edge." *Psychosomatic Medicine* 72.4 (2010): 365. Print.

Laitinen, TT, et al. "Ideal Cardiovascular Health in Childhood and Cardiometabolic Outcomes in Adulthood: The Cardiovascular Risk in Young Finns Study." *Circulation* 125.16 (2012): 1971–1978. Web.

Lange, T, et al. "Sleep Enhances the Human Antibody Response to Hepatitis A Vaccination." *Psychosomatic Medicine* 65 (2003): 831–835.

Lay, CH, and Schouwenburg, HC. "Trait Procrastination, Time Management, and Academic Behavior." *Journal of Social Behavior and Personality* 8 (1993): 647–662.

Lee, Donghyuck, et al. "The Effects of College Counseling Services on Academic Performance and Retention." *Journal of College Student Development* 50.3 (2009): 305–319.

Levine, JA. "Sick of Sitting." *Diabetologia* 58 (2015): 1751–1758.

Linley, PA, Maltby, J, and Proctor, Carmel. "Strengths Use as a Predictor of Well-being and Health-Related Quality of Life." *Journal of Happiness Studies* 12 (2011): 153–169.

Linley, PA, et al. "Using Signature Strengths in Pursuit of Goals: Effects on Goal Progress, Need Satisfaction, and Well-being, and Implications for Coaching Psychologists." *International Coaching Psychology Review* 5.1 (2010): 8–17.

Locke, EA. "Motivation through Conscious Goal Setting." *Applied and Preventative Psychology* 5 (1996): 117–124.

Locke, Edwin A, and Latham, Gary P. "Building a Practically Useful Theory of Goal Setting and Task Motivation: A 35-Year Odyssey." *American Psychologist* 57.9 (2002): 705.

Loehr, James E, and Tony Schwartz. *The Power of Full Engagement: Managing Energy, Not Time, Is the Key to High Performance and Personal Renewal.* New York, NY: Free Press, a division of Simon and Schuster, Inc., 2003. Print.

Logel, Christine, and Cohen, Geoffrey L. "The Role of the Self in Physical Health Testing the Effect of a Values-Affirmation Intervention on Weight Loss." *Psychological Science* 23.1 (2012): 53–55.

Loprenzi, PD, et al. "Physical Activity and the Brain: A Review of this Dynamic, Bi-directional Relationship." *Brain Research* 1539 (2013): 95–104.

Lund, HG, et al. "Sleep Patterns and Predictors of Disturbed Sleep in a Large Population of College Students." *The Journal of Adolescent Health* 46 (2010): 124–132.

Luyster, FS, et al. "Sleep: A Health Imperative." *Sleep* 35 (2012): 727–734.

Macan, TH, et al. "College Students' Time Management: Correlations with Academic Performance and Stress." *Journal of Educational Psychology* 82 (1990): 760.

Manosso, Luana M, Moretti, Morgana, and Rodrigues, Ana Lúcia S. "Nutritional Strategies for Dealing with Depression." *Food & Function* 4.12 (2013): 1776–1793. Print.

Matthews, CE, et al. "Amount of Time Spent in Sedentary Behaviors in the United States, 2003-2004." *American Journal of Epidemiology* 167.7 (2008): 875–881.

Mattson, MP. "Energy Intake and Exercise as Determinants of Brain Health and Vulnerability to Injury and Disease." *Cell Metabolism* 16.6 (2012): 706–722.

McEwen, Bruce S. "Central Effects of Stress Hormones in Health and Disease: Understanding the Protective and Damaging Effects of Stress and Stress Mediators." *European Journal of Pharmacology* 583.2-3 (2008): 174–185. doi:10.1016/j.ejphar.2007.11.071.

Minkel, JD, et al. "Sleep Deprivation and Stressors: Evidence for Elevated Negative Affect in Response to Mild Stressors When Sleep Deprived." *Emotion* 12 (2012): 1015–1020.

Misra, Ranjita, and McKean, Michelle. "College Students' Academic Stress and Its Relation to Their Anxiety, Time Management, and Leisure Satisfaction." *American Journal of Health Studies* 16.1 (2000).

Morisano, Dominique, et al. "Setting, Elaborating, and Reflecting on Personal Goals Improves Academic Performance." *Journal of Applied Psychology* 95.2 (2010): 255–264.

Murphy, Sherry L, Xu, Jiaquan, and Kochanek, Kenneth D, Division of Vital Statistics "BRFSS 2011 Survey Data and Documentation" *National Vital Statistics Reports* 61.4 (2013). Deaths: Final Data for 2010. http://www.cdc.gov/brfss/annual_data/annual_2011.htm.

Niemiec, Ryan M. *Mindfulness and Character Strengths: A Practical Guide to Flourishing*. Boston, MA: Hogrefe, 2014. pp. 26–27. Print.

Ohayon, MM, and Roth, T. "Place of Chronic Insomnia in the Course of Depressive and Anxiety Disorders." *Journal of Psychiatric Research* 37 (2003): 9–15.

Owen, N, et al. "Too Much Sitting: The Population Health Science of Sedentary Behavior." *Exercise and Sport Science Reviews* 38.3 (2010): 105–113.

Palma, JA, Urrestarazu, E, and Iriarte, J. "Sleep Loss as Risk Factor for Neurologic Disorders: A Review." *Sleep Medicine* 14 (2013): 229–236.

Papanikolaou, Z, et al. "The Freshman Experience: High Stress-Low Grades." *Athletic Insight: The Online Journal of Sport Psychology* 5 (2003).

Pearson, Erin S. "Goal Setting as a Health Behavior Change Strategy in Overweight and Obese Adults: A Systematic Literature Review Examining Intervention Components." *Patient Education and Counseling* 87.1 (2012): 32–42. Web.

Park, Nansook, Peterson, Christopher, and Seligman, Martin EP. "Strengths of Character and Well-Being." *Journal of Social and Clinical Psychology* 23.5 (2004): 603–619.

Peterson, C, and Park, N. "Classifying and Measuring Strengths of Character." 2009. *Oxford Handbook of Positive Psychology*. Ed. Shane J. Lopez and C. R. Snyder, 2nd ed. (pp. 25–33). New York, NY: Oxford University Press.

Peterson, C, and Seligman, MEP. *Character Strengths and Virtues: A Handbook and Classification*. New York, NY: Oxford University Press and Washington, DC: American Psychological Association, 2004.

Physical Activity Guidelines Advisory Committee. *Physical Activity Guidelines Advisory Committee Report. Part G. Section 8: Mental Health, 2008*. Washington, DC: US Department of Health and Human Services, Office of Disease Prevention and Health Promotion, 2008. http://www.health.gov/paguidelines/Report/pdf/CommitteeReport.pdf. Web. 14 June 2015.

Raphaely, T, et al. "Flexitarianism (Flexible or Part-Time Vegetarianism): A User-Based Dietary Choice for Improved Well-Being." *International Journal of User-Driven Healthcare (IJUDH)* 3.3 (2013): 40–64.

Ratanasiripong, Paul, et al. "Biofeedback and Counseling for Stress and Anxiety Among College Students." *Journal of College Student Development* 53.5 (2012): 742–749. Article.

Ratey, John J, and Eric Hagerman. *Spark*. New York, NY: Little, Brown, 2008. Print.

Rogatko, TP "The Influence of Flow on Positive Affect in College Students." *Journal of Happiness Studies* 10 (2009): 133–148.

Ruthig, JC, et al. "Changes in College Student Health: Implications for Academic Performance." *College Student Health* 52.3 (2011): 307–320.

Sapolosky, RM. "Why Stress Is Bad for Your Brain." *Science* 273.5276 (1996): 749–750. Web. DOI: 10.1126/science.273.5276.749.

Schwartz, Mark S, and Andrasik, Frank. *Biofeedback: A Practitioner's Guide*. New York, NY: Guilford Press, 2003.

Scullin, MK, and Bliwise, DL. "Sleep, Cognition, and Normal Aging: Integrating a Half Century of Multidisciplinary Research." *Perspectives on Psychological Science* 10 (2015): 97–137.

Seligman, M. *Flourish—A Visionary New Understanding of Happiness and Well-Being.* New York: Free Press, a division of Simon and Schuster, Inc., 2011. Print.

Spiegel, K, et al. "Sleep Loss: A Novel Risk Factor for Insulin Resistance and Type 2 Diabetes." *Journal of Applied Physiology* 99 (2005): 2008–2019.

Spiegel, K, et al. "Brief Communication: Sleep Curtailment in Healthy Young Men Is Associated with Decreased Leptin Levels, Elevated Ghrelin Levels, and Increased Hunger and Appetite." *Annals of Internal Medicine* 141 (2004): 846–850.

"Stress in America℠ Paying with Our Health". American Psychological Association. 2015. www.apa.org/news/press/releases/stress/2014/stress-report.pdf. 4 Feb.

Themanson, JR, Pontifex, MB, and Hillman, CH. "Fitness and Action Monitoring: Evidence for Improved Cognitive Flexibility in Young Adults." *Cognitive Neuroscience* 157.2 (2008): 319–328.

Tudor-Locke, C, et al. "How Many Steps/Day are Enough? For Adults." *International Journal of Behavioral Nutrition and Physical Activity* 8 (2011): 79.

Tudor-Locke, C, et al. "Revisiting "How Many Steps Are Enough?" *Medicine and Science in Sport and Exercise* 40.7 Suppl (2008): S537–S543.

US Department of Health and Human Services. *2008 Physical Activity Guidelines for Americans.* Washington, DC: US Department of Health and Human Services, 2008. http://www.health.gov/paguidelines. 14 June 2015.

Van Dongen, HP, et al. "The Cumulative Cost of Additional Wakefulness: Dose-Response Effects on Neurobehavioral Functions and Sleep Physiology from Chronic Sleep Restriction and Total Sleep Deprivation." *Sleep* 26 (2003): 117–126.

van Praag, H, et al. "Exercise, Energy Intake, Glucose Homeostasis, and the Brain." *The Journal of Neuroscience* 34.46 (2014):15139–15149.

Wagner, U, et al. "Sleep Inspires Insight." *Nature* 427 (2004): 352–355.

Wald, A, et al. "Associations Between Healthy Lifestyle Behaviors and Academic Performance in U.S. Undergraduates: A Secondary Analysis of the American College Health Association's National College Health Assessment II." *American Journal of Health Promotion* 28.5 (2014): 298–305.

Wardlaw, Cheryl. *Taming Stress: The Body's Responses to Life's Demands.* Amazon Digital Services, Inc., 2012. Print.

Walker, MP, et al. "Practice with Sleep Makes Perfect: Sleep-Dependent Motor Skill Learning." *Neuron* 35 (2002a): 205–211.

Walker, MP, et al. "Cognitive Flexibility across the Sleep-Wake Cycle: REM-Sleep Enhancement of Anagram Problem Solving." *Cognitive Brain Research* 14 (2002b): 317–324.

Wood, Alex M, et al. "Using Personal and Psychological Strengths Leads to Increases in Well-Being Over Time: A Longitudinal Study and the Development of the Strengths Use Questionnaire." *Personality and Individual Differences* 50.1 (2011): 15–19. Web.

Xie, L, et al. "Sleep Drives Metabolite Clearance from the Adult Brain." *Science* 342 (2013): 373–377.